T0224975

Rhinosporidiosis

Nitin M. Nagarkar • Rupa Mehta

Editors

Rhinosporidiosis

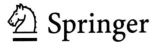 Springer

Editors
Nitin M. Nagarkar
Director
All India Institute of Medical Sciences
Raipur, Chhattisgarh, India

Rupa Mehta
Additional Professor
Department of ENT
All India Institute of Medical Sciences
Raipur, Chhattisgarh, India

ISBN 978-981-16-8510-1   ISBN 978-981-16-8508-8   (eBook)
https://doi.org/10.1007/978-981-16-8508-8

This Springer imprint is published by the registered company Springer Nature Singapore Pte Ltd.
The registered company address is: 152 Beach Road, #21-01/04 Gateway East, Singapore 189721, Singapore

*To my wife Anu and son Rishabh—Pillars of
my strength, for their unconditional love and
support
To my teachers and colleagues, for their faith
and encouragement
To our patients for their trust at all times!
NMN
To my parents and brother Hitesh for their
unending love
To my husband, Harshal and kids—Harshit
and Rupansh for immense support and
understanding
To my teachers, patients and God Almighty
for their constant blessings
RM*

Foreword

"It's a Bird... It's a Plane... It's Superman", the 1966 musical composed by Charles Strouse shows the dilemma in the recognition, nature, and the confusion in the issues of even common objects. It is no surprise then, that despite it being with us for so long, Rhinosporidiosis can still make us say.... "It's a fungus....It's a bacteria...It's a new species...It's....." It's a dilemma. It's an enigma.

Although a large body of literature exists focusing on this problem, this much needed initiative by Prof. Nitin M. Nagarkar and Dr. Rupa Mehta and their colleagues covers the various aspects of the disease which despite the fact that Rhinosporidiosis and its causative pathogen *Rhinosporidium seeberi* have been known to us for over a hundred years, is still an enigma. There are debates surrounding the mode of infection, mechanisms of spread, mechanisms of immunity, and some aspects of histopathology.

Recognizing the importance of increasing the access of knowledge with respect to issues like Rhinosporidiosis, this monograph brings into focus a collection of well researched and documented information about this disease. It is heartening to note that all involved medical streams—basic sciences—microbiology, pathology, epidemiology, pharmacology, and clinical sciences—otorhinolaryngology, ophthalmology, dermatology, and orthopedics have shared their expertise and experience in this monograph to provide a comprehensive overview of this disease entity.

The use of endoscopes has greatly increased the visibility of the lesion and has helped in better evaluation, excision, and detection of recurrence, which is not so uncommon. Coblators and microdebriders are also very useful in surgery for rhinosporidiosis.

As our world continues to generate unimaginable amounts of data, this more data leads to more correlations, and more of such correlations can lead to more discoveries.

Hans Rosling

The work is related not only to some of the unanswered questions, but also to unquestioned answers. We are sure this monograph will have a wide global readership among medical students, postgraduates, and clinicians of all involved specialities.

We heartily wish for more interinstitutional, interdepartmental collaborative research between various countries in which Rhinosporidiosis is endemic.

Suresh C. Sharma
National Medical Commission
New Delhi, India
Department of Otorhinolaryngology
AIIMS
New Delhi, India

Achal Gulati
Maulana Azad Medical College
New Delhi, India

Preface

Rhinosporidiosis affects multiple body parts (nose nasopharynx, oropharynx, oral cavity, eyes skin, bones) and has a very specific geographical regional distribution. Though it has been known for several decades and is a major public health problem in various parts of the world (Sri Lanka, India, Pakistan, Myanmar), yet many unresolved enigmas remain around the various aspects of this disease and its treatment.

Rhinosporidiosis is endemic in central and southern India. Through this monograph, we wish to share our team's experience of managing varied presentations of nose, naso-oropharyngeal, cutaneous, musculoskeletal, and ophthalmic rhinosporidiosis. We have also summarized the basic science—microbiological, pathological, pharmacological, and epidemiological aspects and also the future prospects of research on rhinosporidiosis. Therefore, this monograph will serve as a complete resource for all those who wish to know about this disease entity.

We wish to thank our patients, our fellow colleagues from all the departments, our senior and junior residents, and our family members for supporting us in our endeavor.

Chhattisgarh, India

Nitin M. Nagarkar
Rupa Mehta

Contents

List of Contributors

Alok C. Agrawal Professor & Head, Department of Orthopedics, AIIMS, Raipur, India

Ripu Daman Arora Additional Professor, Department of ENT and Head Neck Surgery, AIIMS, Raipur, India

Sharmistha Chakravarty Assistant Professor, Department of ENT and Head Neck Surgery, AIIMS, Raipur, India

Megha Chandran PG-JR 3, Department of ENT and Head Neck Surgery, AIIMS, Raipur, India

Amit Kumar Chowhan, MD Professor & HOD, Department of Pathology and Laboratory Medicine, AIIMS, Raipur, India

Suryaprakash Dhaneria Professor & HOD, Department of Pharmacology, AIIMS, Raipur, India

Nitin Gaikwad Professor, Department of Pharmacology, AIIMS, Raipur, India

Abhiruchi Galhotra Professor, Department of CFM, AIIMS, Raipur, India

Anjan K. Giri Additional Professor, Department of CFM, AIIMS, Raipur, India

Nighat Hussain, MD Professor, Department of Pathology and Laboratory Medicine, AIIMS, Raipur, India

Bikram Kar Associate Professor, Department of Orthopedics, AIIMS, Raipur, India

Rupa Mehta, MS, DNB, MNAMS Additional Professor, Department of ENT, AIIMS, Raipur, India

Neeta Misra Additional Professor, Department of Ophthalmology, AIIMS, Raipur, India

Somen Misra Professor & HOD, Department of Ophthalmology, AIIMS, Raipur, India

Nitin M. Nagarkar, MS, DNB, MNAMS, FIMSA Director & CEO, Department of ENT and Head Neck Surgery, AIIMS, Raipur, India

Nidhin SB Senior Resident, Department of ENT and Head Neck Surgery, AIIMS, Raipur, India

Srikanta Padhan MPH, Department of CFM, AIIMS, Raipur, India

Neel Prabha Assistant Professor, Department of Dermatology, All India Institute of Medical Sciences, Raipur, India

Harshal Sakale Associate Professor, Department of Orthopedics, AIIMS, Raipur, India

Satish Satpute Assistant Professor, Department of ENT and Head Neck Surgery, AIIMS, Raipur, India

Pranav Sheth PG-JR 3, Department of Pharmacology, AIIMS, Raipur, India

Ambesh Singh, MCH HNSO (S.R.) Mch Head & Neck Surgery & Oncology SR3, Department of ENT and Head Neck Surgery, AIIMS, Raipur, India

Archana Wankhade Additional professor, Department of Microbiology, AIIMS, Raipur, India

Introduction

Sharmistha Chakravarty, Rupa Mehta, and Nitin M. Nagarkar

"Arise, awake and do not stop till the goal is reached"
—*Swami Vivekananda*

Rhinosporidiosis is an archaic disease spanning over centuries and spreading across borders to have a global existence. It is a chronic granulomatous disease that is endemic in South Asian countries like India and Sri Lanka, but cases have been reported from America, Europe and Africa [1]. In the 1890s, an apparent sporozoan parasite was detailed in nasal polyps and was given the nomenclature of *Coccidium seeberia* after the protozoal subdivision Coccidia. Later in the early 1900s, the life cycle of the organism was analyzed and it was argued to be a fungus-like protozoan belonging to the class Mesomycetozoea (between fungi and animals) with a proposed name *Rhinosporidium seeberi* [2, 3]. Thereafter, the microbe has been predominantly classified as a fungus, albeit its debatable taxonomy. There exists alternative hypothesis regarding non-fungal aetiology of this disease, namely, the prokaryotic cyanobacterium, Microcystis aeruginosa, and the proposed theory that *R. seeberi* is related to a group of fish parasites (the DRIP clade: Dermocystidium, Rosette agent, Ichthyophonus and Psorospermium) that flourish in hot and humid climate [4]. Accordingly, coastal areas of the tropics of southern India form the endemic zones with a high rate of prevalence of this disease. The phylogenetic distribution of this group of parasites arises from the observation that they share common features with early diverging animals and fungi. Presence of chitin synthase genes in *Rhinosporidium seeberi* and the ability to produce endosporulating cells in the infected host favoured its existence as fungal pathogen [1].

S. Chakravarty (✉) · R. Mehta · N. M. Nagarkar
Department of ENT and Head Neck Surgery, AIIMS, Raipur, India

© The Author(s), under exclusive license to Springer Nature Singapore Pte Ltd. 2022
N. M. Nagarkar, R. Mehta (eds.), *Rhinosporidiosis*,
https://doi.org/10.1007/978-981-16-8508-8_1

1

Epidemiology

Rhinosporidiosis has a diversified global presence in about 70 countries and the highest incidence has been from India and Sri Lanka. Though most cases of human rhinosporidiosis in Western countries occurred in people who probably acquired the disease in their native lands in Asia, a few cases have been reported in persons who have never travelled to endemic areas. Rhinosporidiosis is an infective disease but not an infectious one, as no transmission has ever been documented of cross-infection between members of the same family or between animals and humans [5]. Majority of cases are sporadic. The exact mode of transmission is ambiguous, though, presumably the disease gets transmitted through infected soil and stagnant water, as contaminated water bodies form the natural aquatic habitat of spores of *Rhinosporidium seeberi*. The route of entry is through the traumatized epithelium, mainly at mucocutaneous junctions. Rural habitat and pond bathing is considered to be an important risk factor that also explains the predeliction of nose, nasopharynx, lacrimal apparatus and conjunctiva as accessible mucosal sites where the organism gains easy portal of entry. Over 70% cases are reported in nasal mucosa and 15% show ocular involvement. The routes of transmission are primarily divided into three categories—autoinoculation as a result of overspill of endospores during surgery [6], haematogenous dissemination [7] and lymphatic spread [8]. Contact with faeces of infected livestock and working in contaminated agricultural fields has also been reported as risk factors. Rhinosporidiosis is more common in younger age groups and amongst males as this group is occupationally active with more outdoor activity [9]. The hot weather in most part of the year, the perpetual habit of pond-bathing due to relative scarcity of clean water in the rural areas, and agriculture being the primary means of livelihood have a huge impact on rising incidence of rhinosporidiosis in India and other South Asian countries.

A pertinent observation in the incidence of this disease is that though a multitude number of people are exposed to contaminated waters, only a few acquire infection and develop progressive disease. This might indicate the existence of predisposing determinants in the host. The possibility of non-specific immune reaction in the host, blood group antigens and variation in HLA types towards pathogenesis of the disease has been considered in a few studies. In India, the highest incidence of rhinosporidiosis was in blood Group O (70%); the next highest incidence was in Group AB though in the general population Group AB is rare [10]. The epidemiology of rhinosporidiosis is still obscure and further investigations are needed to understand whether rhinosporidiosis is acquired in particular communities or if unrecognized factors exist that may explain the emerging epidemiology of this infection. Two dominant factors play a pivotal role in global spread of this disease: increasing need of working population for travel to faraway geographical areas and the ability of these agents to remain dormant for years.

Pathology

This microbe forms rounded sporangia in the submucosal layer which appear as white dots containing daughter sporangiospores. They vary in size from 10 to 200 mm in diameter. Fungal stains like Gomori Methenamine Silver (GMS) and Periodic Acid-Schiff (PAS), as well as with standard Haematoxylin and Eosin (H&E) stain are used for pathological diagnosis. Rhinosporidiosis manifests as tumour-like masses in the form of a friable, vascular, pedunculated or sessile polyp, with a surface studded with tiny white dots due to spores beneath the epithelium, giving a "strawberry-like" appearance usually of the nasal mucosa or less commonly as ocular and conjunctival lesions. Nasopharyngeal polyps are often multilobed and polyps on the face and trunk have verrucous warty appearance, and are either pedunculated or broad-based sessile polyps.

Rhinosporidial granulomas in disseminated cases occur as subcutaneous lumps with unbroken skin. The morphological element of rhinosporidiosis, for which the proposed term is "Electron Dense Body", was earlier termed as spherule [11].

Clinical Features

The clinical presentation in rhinosporidiosis is predominantly in the second and third decade, but few studies have highlighted a bimodal age of distribution, with multiple peaks around 50 years. As the disease has a slow course, lesions may be present for many years before the patients become symptomatic. The site most commonly involved is the upper airway, notably the anterior nares, the nasal cavity—the inferior turbinates, septum and floor. The nasal and nasopharyngeal mucosa traditionally is the favoured site of inoculation in lieu of exposed mucosa with minor epithelial breach at an accessible site. Patients with nasal involvement often have masses leading to nasal obstruction or bleeding due to polyp formation and it can spread to the nasopharynx, oropharynx, lacrimal system, paranasal sinuses and upper respiratory tract (laryngotracheal complex). Rarely, parotid duct involvement has been reported which clinically presents as cheek swelling often confused with mucous retention cyst or ductocoel [12]. Apart from otorhinolaryngologists, this disease is intriguing to dermatologists and ophthalmologists due to the occurrence of granulomas in the skin, subcutaneous tissues and eye. Occasionally, lesions have been associated with other areas in the head and neck region and rarely in urethral, vaginal and rectal sites [13]. Systemic disease is rare but can unfurl as disseminated mucocutaneous, hepatic, renal, pulmonary, splenic or bone lesions [14].

Nasal obstruction was the predominant symptom followed by epistaxis. Epistaxis is an important presenting complaint in rhinosporidiosis along with a slow-growing nasal mass. The clinical hallmark is a reddish polypoid nasal mass with characteristic "white-dots" (the sporangia), with a history of intermittent nose-bleed, in a villager actively engaged in outdoor activities in the field or waterbodies. Pond bathing has been found to be a significant risk factor in literature from the Indian subcontinent. Rhinosporidiosis is notorious for recurrence. Apart from the intraoperative bleeding that obscures the surgeon's view leading to possible overlooking of small residual lesions, it has been hypothesized that spillage of blood at surgery containing *R. seeberi* spores can inoculate virgin sites. Analyzing the recurrence scenario is of prime importance because they not only reduce the burden of healthcare expenditure, but also improvise the patients' quality of life.

Diagnosis

The diagnosis is primarily clinical based on presence of a friable, vascular polypoidal mass with white dots on the surface. It is established by observing the characteristic appearance of the organism in tissue biopsies and CT scans. The gold standard diagnosis of rhinosporidiosis is by histopathology on biopsied or resected specimens, along with a detailed report of the pathogen in its diverse stages. Certain grey areas do exist in the histopathological assessment, most predominant of which is the absence of the Splendore-Hoeppli reaction (antibody-mediated eosinophilic deposit around rhinosporidial bodies), which is well-marked in invasive, classical mycoses [15]. The absence is all the more surprising because rhinosporidial patients show high titres of antirhinosporidial antibodies [16].

Treatment

The mode of treatment is primarily surgical. Total surgical excision with cauterization of the stalk or base of the polyp with electrocautery is the gold standard treatment. Pedunculated polyps allow complete removal while sessile polyps with broad bases of attachment tend to be recurrent due to spillage of endospores on the perioperative surgical site. The study on *Rhinosporidium seeberi* suffered a major setback when it was realized that it cannot be isolated in vitro, impeding its drug sensitivity tests and clinical application trials [17]. Although multiple drug trials with an array of antibacterial and antifungal drugs have been conducted, the only drug which was found to have some anti-rhinosporidial effect is dapsone (4,4-diaminodiphenyl sulphone), which acts by arresting the maturation of the sporangia and promoting fibrosis in the stroma. The need to develop alternate drug therapies to dapsone is of paramount importance as dapsone is known to cause haemolytic reactions in patients with G6PD deficiency. Ironically geographic regions of Southeast Asia share common endemicity to both rhinosporidiosis and G6PD deficiency.

Recent Advances

Fluorescent in situ hybridization techniques (FISH) have supplemented the evidence that the natural habitats of infective spores are water reservoirs and soil contaminated by waste [18]. Studies on the immunology of the developmental stages of *R. seeberi* are scarce. Immuno-electron microscopy was used to demonstrate an antigen with a potential role in the immunology of rhinosporidiosis. This finding raises the possibility of antigenic variation. Another significant revelation is the presence of immunoglobulin-binding proteins in *R. seeberi*, a phenomenon also described in bacteria, which might contribute to immune evasion by this pathogen [18]. Certain controversial domains that require future research are the factors affecting chronicity, recurrence and dissemination. Rhinosporidiosis is an enigmatic disease with many controversial nuances and increasingly global spread. Adequate research to explain its pathogenesis and treatment strategies shall act as torchbearers to aid in improved patient outcome and overall social well-being as it affects the most productive age group of our society.

References

1. Arseculeratne SN, Ajello L. Rhinosporidium seeberi. In: Hay RJ, Ajello L, editors. Topley & Wilson's Microbiology & Microbial Infections, vol. 4, medical mycology. 9th ed. London: Edward Arnold; 1998. p. 595–615.
2. Herr RA, Ajello L, Taylor JW, Arseculeratne SN, Mendoza L. Phylogenetic analysis of *Rhinosporidium seeberi*'s 18S small-subunit ribosomal DNA groups this pathogen among members of the protistan mesomycetozoa clade. J Clin Microbiol. 1999;37:2750–4.
3. Ajello L, Mendoza L. The phylogeny of *Rhinosporidium seeberi*. 14th Meeting of the International Society for Human and Animal Mycology. Buenos Aires, Argentina, 2000: 78.
4. Ragan MA, Goggin CL, Cawthorn RJ, et al. A novel clade of protistan parasites near the animal-fungal divergence. Proc Natl Acad Sci U S A. 1996;93:11907–12.
5. Arseculeratne SN. Recent advances in Rhinosporidiosis and *Rhinosporidium seeberi*. Indian J Med Microbiol. 2002;20(3):119–31.
6. Capoor MR, Khanna G, Rajni, et al. Rhinosporidiosis in Delhi, North India: case series from a non-endemic area and mini-review. Mycopathologia. 2008;168:89–94.
7. Rajam RV, Viswanathan GC. Rhinosporidiosis: a study with a report of a fatal case with systemic dissemination. Ind J Surg. 1955;17:269–98.
8. Ashworth JH. On *Rhinosporidium seeberi* (Wernicke, 1903) with special reference to its sporulation and affinities. Trans Roy Soc Edinburg. 1923;53:301–42.
9. Makannavar JH, Chavan SS. Rhinosporidiosis—a clinicopathological study of 34 cases. Indian J Pathol Microbiol. 2001;44:17–21.
10. Kameswaran S, Lakshmanan M. Rhinosporidiosis. In: Kameswaran S, Kameswaran M, editors. ENT disorders in a tropical environment. Chennai: MERF Publications; 1999. p. 19–34.
11. Kennedy FA, Buggage RR, Ajello L. Rhinosporidiosis: a description of an unprecedented outbreak in captive swans *(Cygnus* spp.) and a proposal for revision of the ontogenic nomenclature of *Rhinosporidium seeberi*. J Med Vet Mycol. 1995;37:157–65.
12. Samal S, Pradhan P, Preetam C. Isolated primary Rhinosporidiosis of the parotid duct: a rare presentation. Iran J Otorhinolaryngol. 2020;32(3):193–6. https://doi.org/10.22038/ijorl.2020.43051.2408.

13. Pal DK, Moulik D, Chowdhury MK. Genitourinary rhinosporidiosis. Indian J Urol. 2008;24:419–21.
14. Ho MS, Tay BK. Disseminated rhinosporidiosis. Ann Acad Med Singapore. 1986;15:80–3.
15. Arseculeratne SN, Atapattu DN, Rajapakse RPVJ, Balasooriya P, Fernando R, Wijewardena T. The humoral immune response in human rhinosporidiosis. Proc Kandy Soc Med. 1999;21:9.
16. Hutt MSR, Fernandes BJ, Templeton AC. Myospherulosis (Subcutaneous Spherulocystic Disease). Trans Roy Soc Trop Med Hyg. 1971;65:182–188.
17. Ahluwalia KB. New interpretations in rhinosporidiosis, enigmatic disease of the last nine decades. J Submicrosc Cytol Pathol. 1992;24:109–14.
18. Kaluarachchi K, Sumathipala S, Eriyagama N, Atapattu D, Arseculeratne S. The identification of the natural habitat of *Rhinosporidium seeberi* with *Rhinosporidium seeberi*—specific *in situ* hybridization probe *s*. J Infect Dis Antimicrob Agents. 2008;25:25–32.

Epidemiology of Rhinosporidiosis

Anjan K. Giri, Srikanta Padhan, and Abhiruchi Galhotra

Introduction

Rhinosporidiosis is a chronic granulomatous infective, non-contagious, sporadic, benign, usually non-fatal disorder producing polypoidal, pedunculated, and soft tissue mass [1]. It is a chronic condition that frequently recurs after surgery and occasionally spreads from the initial focus, which is usually observed in the upper respiratory tract. More than 70% of cases affect the nose and the nasopharynx. Ocular lesions, particularly of the conjunctiva and lachrymal sac, account for 15% of cases. Rhinosporidial polyps are also reported from different rare sites like lips, palate, uvula, maxillary antrum, epiglottis, larynx, trachea, bronchus, ear, scalp, vulva, penis, rectum, or skin. Infections that spread to the limbs, trunk, bone, brain, and internal organs have been documented [2, 3].

The aetiological agent of Rhinosporidiosis is *Rhinosporidium Seeberi* has been an enigma for a century. The causal pathogen is commonly assumed to be a fungus; however, its specific taxonomy is still being debated [4]. Guillermo Seeber reported Rhinosporidiosis for the first time in 1900 from the new world city of Buenos Aires, Argentina. It appeared as a nasal polyp, and Seeber rightly thought that the condition was caused by an infection. He proposed the infective aetiology for this disease to be a fungus, which was later isolated by Ashworth in 1923, who in turn described the life cycle of the organism and established the nomenclature *Rhinosporidium seeberi* [5]. Rhinosporidiosis was later discovered in both the new and the old worlds.

In India, the first case was reported by O'Kinealy in 1903, which was observed by him in 1894. Rhinosporidiosis is a sporing organism, and Kannankutty first identified its life cycle in 1974. He showed that Rhinosporidiosis produces a chemical comparable to hyaluronidase that causes submucosal dissemination [6].

A. K. Giri · S. Padhan · A. Galhotra (✉)
Department of CFM, AIIMS, Raipur, India
e-mail: abhiruchigalhotra@aiimsraipur.edu.in

© The Author(s), under exclusive license to Springer Nature Singapore Pte Ltd. 2022
N. M. Nagarkar, R. Mehta (eds.), *Rhinosporidiosis*,
https://doi.org/10.1007/978-981-16-8508-8_2

Human beings are not the only definitive host for the organism. A wide range of domestic and wild animals, including cows, buffaloes, dogs, cats, horses, mules, ducks, and swans, are also found to be affected [7].

Problem/Prevalence

World

Rhinosporidiosis has been recorded in around 70 countries, with a wide range of geographical distribution and clinical manifestations. Although the disease is sporadic in parts of Europe, Africa, the southern United States, North, and South American temperate regions, as well as western and Middle Eastern countries, it is endemic in tropical areas, such as Brazil, Argentina, Uganda, Texas, India, and Sri Lanka [8, 9]. The disease can be distributed in a large scale due to trading, international import, intercontinental movement of affected animals or human beings.

Southeast Asia

Rhinosporidiosis is most prevalent in South Asia, particularly in southern India and Sri Lanka. Increased migration to the West of people who contracted Rhinosporidiosis in their original Asian countries has led to an increase in the disease's incidence in the West. However, 90% of the total cases were found to be present in the Indian Subcontinent [10].

India

Bihar was the first state in India to register a Rhinosporidiosis. It has been reported in Madhya Pradesh, Maharashtra, Odisha, Pondicherry, Rajasthan, Uttar Pradesh, Haryana, Kerala, Tamil Nadu, West Bengal, and Chhattisgarh [11]. The disease is quite common in Raipur, Durg, Bilaspur, and Dhamtari districts of Chhattisgarh State [12].

Epidemiology

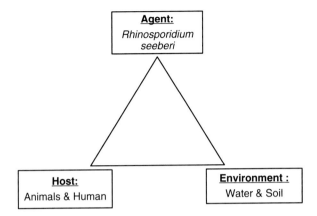

Fig. 1 An epidemiological triad of Rhinosporidiosis

Agent

Rhinosporidium seeberi was once thought to be a sporozoan, but it is now thought to be a fungus, and Ashworth has tentatively placed it in the Olipidiaceae family, order chritridiales of phycomyetes. It is now classified as part of the DRIP clade (Dermocystidium, Rosette agent, Icthyophonus, and Psoropermium), a group of fish parasites that flourish in the hot and humid climate [13]. Despite substantial research, no consensus exists on where Rhinosporidium should be classified in the Taxonomic classification. Even after using sensitive methods such as polymerase chain reactions, it has been impossible to detect fungal proteins in Rhinosporidium.

The infectious agent forms round and thick-walled sporangia in the submucosa of the affected site, varying from 10 to 200 mm in size, which are visible as white dots in the mucosa containing smaller 'daughter cells' (called 'sporangiospores'). It can be visualized with fungal stains such as Gomori Methenamine Silver (GMS) and Periodic Acid-Schiff (PAS), as well as with standard Haematoxylin and Eosin (H&E) staining [14].

Host

Rhinosporidiosis mainly affects mammals, primarily humans, although it has also been observed in domestic and wild animals and birds, including cattle, equines, caprines, dogs, felines, and avian species such as waterfowl, swans, geese, and wild ducks. The disease has also been observed in fish [15–17]. The disease rarely affects children; it is most commonly found in individuals aged 20–40 years for unknown reasons. The disease has also been observed to affect animals such as cows, bulls, horses, mules, and dogs in areas where men and animals share infected ponds [18].

Risk Factors

- **Gender: Male.**
  The study reveals that Rhinosporidiosis is more common in males with a male-to-female ratio of 4:1. This may partly be explained by the lesser chances of animal contact of females and less frequent pond baths [19]. The effect of oestrogens in females might provide some protection from the disease [20].
- **Age: 21–40.**
  According to the available literature, nasal Rhinosporidiosis is most commonly reported in people in their second and third decades, when they are most likely to engage in outdoor activities. Rhinosporidiosis appears to primarily affect young adults in their most productive years. The majority of lesions documented in the third decade of life are at extra nasal locations [21].
- **Bathing History: Ponds.**
  People who bathe in ponds, lakes, or reservoirs are more likely to get rhinosporidiosis of the upper respiratory tract and eye than those who bathe in well water or home tap water. Bathing in rivers with suspended sharp spicules formed from sand may explain the prevalence of ocular lesions in people who are occupationally or recreationally exposed to river water [22].
- **Occupation: Agriculture.**
  Rhinosporidiosis is widespread among farmers who are exposed to dust and muddy water containing soil particles during cultivation. Rhinosporidiosis in the respiratory tract is due to a contaminated wet environment, and that in the ocular form is mainly due to a contaminated dry, dusty environment. The significance of paddy fields as *R. Seeber* sources has probably been overstated [23].
- **Low Socioeconomic status, Rural Residential Status and Backward Caste.**
  The probable reason for this may be the practice of pond bathing and the poorer standards of hygiene among people of low socioeconomic status, rural residential status, and backward class [24].
- **Religion:**

Customs, ways, manners, and sanitary conditions have been found to be associated with the disease incidence [25–27]. However no particular pattern with any community is seen.

- **Blood groups: O.**

ABO blood grouping of the patients reveals that the highest incidence of Rhinosporidiosis is in group O [28].

Environment

The exact mode(s) of transmission and the host or natural reservoirs are unknown; however, the disease is most likely transmitted by infected soil and stagnant water. The disease is spread via water and dust in the environment. Patients with Rhinosporidiosis report bathing in dirty water, contaminated ponds, tanks, and rivers. Sugarcane and paddy producers have reported a high prevalence. The sickness primarily affects those who live near farms and ponds [6, 21].

Modes of Transmission

R. seeberi is a naturally occurring dweller of contaminated water and dust particles that contain spores. The spores of these diseases are found in soil and water, and hence water and soil serve as reservoirs for this pathogen [29]. Contaminated drinking water may expose the nasal mucosa to infection (70% cases). Dust fomites may give rise to ocular form (15%) of disease. It is neither contagious nor transmitted through sexual contact.

The incubation period is very long. Cases are more frequently observed in communities residing near swamp areas as contaminated water serves as a source of infection; hence earlier, it was considered an aquatic fungus. It suggests a possible synergism between aquatic microorganisms and *Rhinosporidium seeberi* for the propagation of infection through stagnant water. Although no direct transmission between humans and animals has been observed, the transmission may occur by direct contact with fungal spores via aerosols, inhalation of dust particles, infected clothing, or swimming in torpid polluted water [30].

Autoinoculation through transepithelial infection, lymphatic and hematogenous pathways into broken skin, or traumatized epithelium may also play a role in the entry and dispersion of spores in the body. Adjacent epithelium may be autoinoculated if endospores can break out of polyps after any trauma or operation. Haematogenous dissemination from a subclinical form of upper respiratory infection (nasal or nasopharynx) can be a possible route of transmission for anatomically distant places in the body of the host. Though few researchers have suggested the probability of lymphatic spread into regional parts of the body but this route is yet not confirmed [31].

Signs and Symptoms

Rhinosporidiosis is painless and not life threatening. Infections of up to 30 years in duration have been reported. The main effects are discomfort when the lesion becomes large enough to obstruct a passage or put pressure on the nerve or vascular tracts. Symptoms vary according to the stage of development and site of infection. The infection produces a slow-growing mass that degenerates into polyps. The polyps are pink to purple, friable, with grey, white, or yellow sporangia on their surface. In the early stages, the patient may complain of nasal discharge, which is often blood-tinged and nasal stuffiness. Sometimes, frank epistaxis is the only presenting complaint [32, 33].

Management

The mainstay of treatment is surgical excision of the lesion. Recurrences are common, and the only drug useful in reducing recurrence is Dapsone which arrests the maturation of sporangia and promotes fibrosis in the stroma when used as an adjunct to surgery, but it has a limited role in reducing the chances of recurrence [34]. Wide surgical excision that is advised cannot be done in most cases because it can result in complications such as septal perforation, excessive crusting, atrophic rhinitis, and haemorrhage. Total excision of the lesion, followed by electrocautery of the base, is the recommended mode of treatment [35]. Recurrence may occur due to spillage of endospores in the surrounding mucosa during removal. Good results without recurrence have been reported following the use of endoscopes during surgery [36].

Prevention and Control

Rhinosporidiosis is an infective condition that is commonly seen in the second and third decades of life. It is seen in people belonging to the low socioeconomic group and those living in rural areas, being more common in males, in individuals who take baths in surface water bodies. In most cases, lesions of Rhinosporidiosis are restricted to the nasal cavity and present with nasal complaints such as nasal mass, nasal bleeding, and nasal obstruction. Nasal endoscopy has to be done in all the suspected cases to detect the site of attachment and the number of lesions. Laryngoscopy is advised in order to rule out the lesions in larynx and laryngopharynx. Surgical excision with electrocautery of the base is preferred to reduce recurrence.

Repeated follow-up of the patients for early detection of lesions is essential. Certain precautions, like avoidance of the use of surface water for bathing and other domestic purposes, also helps in reducing the chances of recurrence. Common water sources used for the bathing of cattle and for human needs should be discouraged. In general, improvement in sanitation and general hygiene, provision of clean water supply, along with imparting proper health education to the high-risk groups residing in rural areas of coastal India can reduce the incidence of Rhinosporidiosis.

The disease incidence may be reduced through raising knowledge on its various mechanisms of transmission, prominent symptoms, early care, and prevention. The role of health care workers has to be emphasized to educate the vulnerable population to modify their risky habits related to their livelihood and lifestyle. A robust system of public health education may help to reduce the incidence of disease.

Contents of Public Health Education

It covers every aspect of personal, family, community, and environmental health.

1. **Personal Health:**

    (i) Maintenance of personal hygiene will be the best option to be safe from an infective disease like Rhinosporidiosis as the disease takes a chronic course which makes diagnosis difficult.

    (ii) Hence swimmers and persons who are frequent visitors to water bodies should have safety precautions as this disease-causing organism gets transferred through cut wounds.

2. **Family Health:**

    (i) Rhinosporidiosis is not contagious. So, there is no transmission of disease among family members. Most probably, the contact of the traumatized epithelium of nostrils with natural aquatic habitat act as the primary mode of entry of pathogen.

    (ii) The role of the family in health promotion and in the prevention of this disease, early diagnosis, and care of the sick is of crucial importance. One of the main tasks of health education is to promote a family's self-reliance, especially regarding the family's responsibilities in maintaining a clean and hygienic environment and in influencing their children to adopt a healthy and hygienic lifestyle.

    (iii) All the family members of endemic villages have a common habit of frequent pond baths. As contaminated water bodies could be the source of infection, hence avoiding water bodies with spores will help to reduce the high incidence of this disease in the villages.

3. **Community Health:**

    (i) The sources of Rhinosporidiosis cases area-wise should be mapped out, which may be helpful to identify the villages with a higher incidence of the disease.

(ii) Health talks regarding symptomatology, disease course, and preventive measures should be given in these villages.

4. **Environmental Health:**

   (i) A health education component should be included in an environmental sanitation program with a focus on clean and safe use of water bodies. It is insufficient to provide sanitary wells, latrines, and waste disposal facilities. If people do not use the facilities, they will continue to suffer from diseases caused by inadequate sanitation.

   (ii) People will participate in identifying their sanitation problems and choosing the remedies and facilities they want if a health education approach is used.

5. **Disease prevention and control.**

   (i) Drugs or surgery alone will not solve health problems without public health education, a person may fall sick again and again from the same disease.

   (ii) Education of the people about the prevention and control of locally endemic diseases is one of the eight essential elements in primary health care.

6. **Use of health services.**

   (i) Many people, particularly in rural areas, do not know what health services are available in their community for Rhinosporidiosis, and many more do not know what signs to look for that indicate a visit to the doctor is necessary.

   (ii) One of the declared aims of public health education is to inform the people about the health services that are available in the community and how they can utilize them.

Approach in Public Health Education

Since individuals vary so much in their socioeconomic conditions, traditions, attitudes, beliefs, and level of knowledge, a single approach may not be suitable. A combination of approaches must be evolved depending upon the local circumstances.

1. **Service approach:**

   (i) It should aim at providing all the health services needed by the people at their doorsteps on the assumption that people would use them to improve their own health.

   (ii) Availability of alternate sources of water for bathing can make people stay away from the contaminated ponds and diseases acquired by it.

2. **Health Education approach:**

   (iii) Because attitudes and behavioural habits are formed in childhood, we need to go back in time and begin health education with young people. The belief is that young people's behaviour is easier to regulate or develop than that of adults.

3. **Primary health care approach:**

(iv) Recurrences are prevalent, most likely due to incomplete excision or intra-operative contamination of neighbouring tissues or cells with resident endo-spores, making the disease much worse. As a future preventive step, electrocauterization at the excision site is indicated.

(v) Newer assays should thus be developed to detect this disease early in human and animal conditions in order to successfully control the disease.

References

1. Sengupta S, Pal S, Biswas BK, Jana S, Biswas S, Minz RS. Clinico-pathological study of 273 cases of Rhinosporidiosis over a period of ten years in a tertiary care institute catering predominantly rural population of tribal origin. Bangladesh Journal of Medical Science. 2015 Apr 18;14(2):159–64.
2. Franca GV Jr, Gomes CC, Sakano E, Altermani AM, Shimizu LT. Nasal rhinosporidiosis in children. J Pedatr (Rio J). 1994;70:299–301.
3. Makannavar JH, Chavan SS. Rhinosporidiosis, a clinicopathological study of 34 cases. Indian J Pathol Microbiol. 2001 Jan 1;44(1):17–21.
4. Arseculeratne SN. Recent advances in rhinosporidiosis and Rhinosporidium seeberi. Indian J Med Microbiol. 2002 Jul 1;20(3):119–31.
5. Ahluwalia KB. New interpretations in rhinosporidiosis, enigmatic disease of the last nine decades. J Submicrosc Cytol Pathol. 1992 Jan 1;24(1):109–14.
6. Banjare B, Sherwani N, Neralwar A. A study on Rhinosporidiosis cases attending a tertiary care hospital of Raipur City (C.G.) India. Indian J Research. 2015;4(8):260–4.
7. Vukovic Z, Bobic-Radovanovic A, Latkovic Z, Radovanovic Z. An epidemiological investigation of the first outbreak of rhinosporidiosis in Europe. J Trop Med Hyg. 1995 Oct 1;98(5):333–7.
8. Rao PR, Jain SN, Rao TH. Animal rhinosporidiosis in India with case reports. Annals of the Belgian society of. Trop Med. 1975;55:119–24.
9. Londero AT, Santos MN, Freitas CJ. Animal rhinosporidiosis in Brazil. Report of three additional cases. Mycopathologia. 1977 Jan 1;60(3):171–3.
10. Morelli L, Polce M, Piscioli F, Del Nonno F, Covello R, Brenna A, et al. Journal search results. Diagn Pathol. 2006;1(1):25.
11. Andleigh HS. Two rare cases of fungus infection of skin in Rajasthan: actinomycosis and rhinosporidiosis. Indian Med Gaz. 1951 Mar;86(3):100.
12. Gupta RK, Singh BP, Singh BR. Rhinosporidiosis in Central India: a cross-sectional study from a tertiary care hospital in Chhattisgarh. Trop Parasitol. 2020 Jul;10(2):120.
13. Das C, Das SK, Chatterjee P, Bandyopadhyay SN. Series of atypical Rhinosporidiosis: our experience in Western part of West Bengal. Indian J Otolaryngol Head Neck Surg. 2019 Nov;71(3):1863–70.
14. Pandey RK, Kumar A, Kumar D. Incidence of Rhinosporidiosis in Jharkhand. & Chao SS, Loh KS. Rhinosporidiosis: an unusual cause of nasal masses gains prominence. Singap Med J. 2004 May 1;45:224–6.
15. Myers DD, Simon J, Case MT. Rhinosporidiosis in a horse. J Am Vet Med Assoc. 1964;145(4):345–7.

16. Pal M. Nasal rhinosporidiosis in a bullock in Gujarat (India). Rev Iberoam Micol. 1995;12(3):61–2.
17. Das S, Kashyap B, Barua M, Gupta N, Saha R, Vaid L, Banka A. Nasal rhinosporidiosis in humans: new interpretations and a review of the literature of this enigmatic disease. Med Mycol. 2011 Apr 1;49(3):311–5.
18. Dhingra P, Dhingra S. Diseases of ear, nose and throat & head and neck surgery. 6th ed. New Delhi: Elsevier; 2014.
19. Chao SS, Loh KS. Rhinosporidiosis: an unusual cause of nasal masses gains prominence. Singap Med J. 2004 May 1;45:224–6.
20. Venkateswaran S, Date A, Job A, Mathan M. Light and electron microscopic findings in rhino-sporidiosis after dapsone therapy. Tropical Med Int Health. 1997 Dec;2(12):1128–32.
21. Dutta S, Haldar D, Dutta M, Barik S, Biswas KD, Sinha R. Socio-demographic correlates of rhinosporidiosis: a hospital-based epidemiologic study in Purulia, India. Indian J Otolaryngol Head Neck Surg. 2017 Mar 1;69(1):108–12.
22. Senaratne T, Senanayake S, Edussuriya K, Wijenayake P, Arseculeratne S. Ocular Rhinosporidiosis with staphyloma formation: the first report in Sri Lanka. J Infect Dis Antimicrob Agents. 2007;24:133–41.
23. Karunaratne WA, Rhinosporidiosis in Man. Rhinosporidiosis in Man. Athlone: University of London; 1964.
24. Pandey RK, Kumar A, Kumar D. Incidence of Rhinosporidiosis in Jharkhand. Indian J Pathol Microbiol. 2001;44(1):17–21.
25. Kurup PK. Rhinosporidium kinealyi infection. Indian Med Gaz. 1931 May;66(5):239.
26. Arseculeratne SN, Sumathipala S, Eriyagama NB. Patterns of Rhinosporidiosis in Sri Lanka: comparison with international data. Southeast Asian J Trop Med Public Health. 2010 Jan 1;41(1):175.
27. Kutty MK, Unni PN. Rhinosporidiosis of the urethra. A case report. Trop Geogr Med. 1969;21(3):338–40.
28. Jain SN. Aetiology and incidence of rhinosporidiosis. Indian J Otolaryngol. 1967 Mar 1;19(1):1–21.
29. Rath R, Baig SA, Debata T. Rhinosporidiosis presenting as an oropharyngeal mass: a clinical predicament? J Nat Sci Biol Med. 2015 Jan;6(1):241.
30. Govinda R, Lakshminarayana CS. Investigation into transmission, growth and serology in rhinosporidiosis. Indian J Med Res. 1962;50(3):363–70.
31. Vanbreuseghem R. Rhinosporidiosis: clinical aspects, epidemiology and ultrastructural studies on Rhinosporidium seeberi. Dermatol Monatsschr. 1976 Jun 1;162(6):512–26.
32. Vadakkan JR, Ganeshbala A, Jalagandesh B. A clinical study of rhinosporidiosis in rural coastal population: our experience. J Evol Med Dent Sci. 2014 Oct 9;3(51):11938–43.
33. Rippon JW. Medical mycology; the pathogenic fungi and the pathogenic actinomycetes. Eastbourne: UK; WB Saunders Company; 1982.
34. Branscomb R. Rhinosporidiosis update. Lab Med. 2002 Aug 1;33(8):631–3.
35. Sarker MM, Kibria AG, Haque MM. Disseminated subcutaneous rhinosporidiosis: a case report. TAJ: J Teach Assoc. 2006;19(1):31–3.
36. Sonkhya N, Singhal P, Mishra P. Naso-oropharyngeal rhinosporidiosis: endoscopic removal. Indian J Otolaryngol Head Neck Surg. 2005 Oct;57(4):354–6.

Microbiological Aspect of Rhinosporidiosis

Archana Wankhade

Introduction

Rhinosporidiosis is a disease caused by *Rhinosporidium seeberi*, which is occurring universally excluding Australia. It endemic in India and Sri Lanka [1]. Contrasting with other infectious diseases which can be identified and characterized easily, there are still many basic issues concerning with pathogen and disease which is not solved completely till date. In this script taxonomy, morphology, life cycle, transmission and ecological sources have been mentioned.

Classification:

- Kingdom—Protozoa
- Sub-kingdom—Neozoa
- Infra-kingdom—Neomonada
- Phylum—Neomonada
- Subphylum—Mesomycetozoa
- (Formerly Ichthyosporea)
- Class—Mesomycetozoea
- Order—Dermocystida
- Family—Rhinosporideaceae
- (Mendoza et al. 2002)
- Dermocystidium spp.
- Rhinosporidium seeberi

A. Wankhade (✉)
Department of Microbiology, AIIMS, Raipur, India

© The Author(s), under exclusive license to Springer Nature Singapore Pte Ltd. 2022
N. M. Nagarkar, R. Mehta (eds.), *Rhinosporidiosis*,
https://doi.org/10.1007/978-981-16-8508-8_3

17

The *Mesomycetozoa* is a small group of pathogens associated with aquatic habitats, phylogenetically located between animals and fungi. They have endospore-like parasitic stages and cannot be grown on artificial media [2]. The taxonomical journey is mentioned below.

Taxonomy

Due to the absence of pure isolates of the organism due to its difficulty to culture many changes are happened in taxonomy. Previously *R. seeberi* was classified as a sporozoon, then as a phycomycete, and later on it was put in an orphanage of anomalous fungal and fungal-like organisms, and even as a cyanobacterium.

Fredricks et al. described Phylogenetic analysis of the organisms based on 18S SSU rDNA, classified R. seeberi in a new clade which they named the Mesomycetozoea. This new group includes fish and amphibian pathogens in the former DRIP clade (Dermocystidium, the rosette agent, Ichthyophonus, and Psorospermium) [3].

Silva et al. worked on the internal transcribed spacer 1 (ITS1), 5.8S, and ITS2 from eight humans, two swans, and a dog with rhinosporidiosis and were sequenced. The amplification of ITS regions was done with PCR using a primer designed from a unique region of R. seeberi's 18S SSU rRNA genes with the ITS4. ITS4 and ITS 5, the universal primers were also used. Differences in the numbers of nucleotides among strains of Human, swans, and the dog R. seeberi's were observed with ITS sequences. Parsimony analysis strongly suggested that the genus Rhinosporidium may possess multiple host-specific strains [4].

The various developments regarding Rhinopridiosis are mentioned in literature is started in 1892 by Malbran who detected the organism in a nasal polyp and regarded it as a sporozoon, findings remained unpublished [2]. In year 1900, Seeber described the organism (cysts, spores containing "sporozoites") and allied to the Polysporea of the Coccidia, but the organism was nameless and Wernicke termed the organism as Rhinosporidium seeberi [5]. A nasal polyp and its histology (Cyst with a pore, filled with sporules) was described by Vaughan and O'Kinealy. Belou et al. described the organism under the name Coccidium seeberia Wernicke in year 1900. Later on, in year 1904 Minchin and Fantham after studied rhinosporidial tissue and O'Kinealy's named the organism Rhinosporidium kinealyi [2]. Seeber endorsed the generic name Rhinosporidium of Minchin and Fantham, and the specific name seeberi of Wernicke, and established the identity of R. kinealyi with R. seeber in 1912 [5]. Zschokke noticed nasal growth with a similar organism in a horse and named it Rhinosporidium equi [5]. Ciferri et al. in 1936 recognized the identity of R. seeberi and R. equi [2, 6].

Lifecycle of R. seeberi was studied by Ashworth and concluded that the organism is not a fungus but a lower order fungus belonging to class Phycomycetes is also presented by Ashworth in 1923 [7]. Later in 1936, he also concluded that all examples of Rhinosporidium recorded from humans appear to be preferable to one species.

Ashworth (1923) [7] opinions as fungus are based on the following criteria:

1. In the tropic phase, the nutritive reserves are largely the fatty material in fungi.
2. Repeated nuclear division takes place preparatory to the formation of spores and nuclei undergoes mitosis simultaneously a feature more characteristic of lower fungi than of protozoa.
3. Division of cytoplasm occurs without any residual cytoplasm and at a late stage namely after 12 nuclear divisions. After formation of cell, it undergoes divisions to form the spores.
4. The presence of mucoid substance is a common feature of sporangia of fungi.
5. The wall of the sporozoan has no cellulose at any stage and sporangium is made up of cellulose.
6. The development of a pore for the exit of the spores is present in several fungi.

Cariniet et al. described cysts with spores in skin nodules in frogs and created a new genus Dermosporidium for the organism, which he regarded as having close affinities with, but different from, R. seeberi [6].

Vanbreusegham et al. opined that the Rhinosporidium seeberi could be an alga [8].

As it could not be cultivated, the observation were based on electrom microscopy:

1. Like alga, the sporangium walls have chitin externally and hemicellulose internally.
2. There are no chloroplasts as in parasitic algae.
3. The spherules could be developed in chloroplasts.
4. Spherules have DNA.
5. Presence of dictyosome which is absent in many fungi.

Ahluwalia K et al., however, restudied the etiology of the agent producing Rhinosporidiosis. Based on electron microscopy and cytochemical studies, she opined that the sporangium is found to be a unique body containing the residue-loaded lysosomal bodies (spores) for elimination from the system. It is concluded that Rhinosporidiosis is a complex phenotype having unique features in medical fields [9].

Morphology

In the twentieth century, Fredricks et al. in the molecular work amplified a portion of the R. seeberi 18S rRNA gene directly from tissue with polymerase chain reaction (PCR). On the basis of analysis of the aligned sequences and inference of phylogenetic relationships resolved that R. seeberi may be a protist from a completely unique clade of parasites that infect fish and amphibians. In the other tissues infected with R. seeberi found this unique 18S rRNA sequence by Fluorescence in situ hybridization and R. seeberi-specific PCR and concluded that R. seeberi is not a classic fungus, but rather the first known human pathogen from the DRIPs clade, a novel clade of aquatic protistan parasites [3].

Thus, the basis of Molecular biological techniques, demonstrated this organism to be an aquatic protistan parasite, and it placed into a new class, the Mesomycetozoea, along with organisms that also cause similar infections in amphibians and fish [3, 10, 11].

It has two orders Dermocystida and Ichthyophonida. Rhinosporidiosis seeberi is placed in order Dermocystida, previously orphaned aquatic microbes, located at the divergence between animals and fungi. More information about mesomycetozoeans is provided in the review by Mendoza et al. (2002) [11].

The absence of a method to observe the in vitro progress of *R. seeberi* growth there is a paucity of data on the biology of *R. seeberi*.

In literature on rhinosporidiosis found various terms for morphological elements like electron-dense bodies which were termed earlier as spherule, electron-dense circular structure, protrusion of cell wall, electron-dense inclusions, germinative bodies sporozoites, spores, spherules, and spherical bodies. Kennedy et al. (1995) described the new terminologies for the description of various stages of organisms in the tissues [12].

The earlier terminologies and newer terminologies for developemental stages of the organism are described in Table 3.1.

Table 3.1 Various terminologies to describe the developemental stages of the organisms

Earlier terminology	New terminology
Spore, immature spore, endospore, sporoblast, early trophic stage, spherule, conidium, sporule	⟶ Immature endospore
Mature spore, sporont, pansporoblast, merozoite, yeast phase in tissue, spore morula	⟶ Mature endospore
Trophocyte (early, intermediate, late), trophic stage, trophozoite, immature sporangium, granular stage, sporocyst, cyst, spherule, sporangium	⟶ Juvenile sporangium
Endosporulating stage, sporulation phase, trophic sporangium	⟶ Intermediate sporangium
Mature trophocyte, mature cyst, endosporulating stage, adult stage	⟶ Mature sporangium
Intracytoplasmic structures in juvenile sporangium Lipid droplets	⟶ Lipid bodies
Multilamellar bodies	⟶ Laminated bodies
Intracytoplasmic structures in mature endospore	
Lipid bodies, cytoplasmic vacuoles	⟶ Lipid globules
Spherules, electron-dense circular structures, protrusions of cell wall, electron-dense inclusions, germinative bodies, sporozoites, spores, sporules, spherical bodies, spore morulae	⟶ Electron-dense bodies

Biology

Developmental stages of R. seeberi in rhinosporidial to the inner aspect of the sporangial wall are described below [2].

Ontogenic stages of R. seeberi are described on the basis of light microscopical and ultrastructural features of the organism in rhinosporidial tissues of humans and animals, which was uniformly found by many authors.

All the developmental stages were identified on the basis of H & E staining of the rhinosporidial tissue. The "life cycle" of R. seeberi, is presumed from histopathological appearances as the organism is non cultivable.

Trophocyte—These are the immature sporangia. It is 10–100 μm in diameter with refractile eosinophilic walls of thickness 2–3 μm. It contains granular or flocculent cytoplasm and a round, pale nucleus with a prominent nucleolus or karyosome. The wall of it is ~5 microns thick during the young developing stage but becomes thinner at maturity thereby pore is formed. Tropocyte is readily seen with H&E but do not stain well with GMS.

Mature sporangia—These are thick walled (5 μm wide), round, large (100–350 μm in diameter; most commonly 100–200 μm), and contain numerous sporangiospores (endospores) that range from 1 to 10 μm in diameter. The wall of mature sporangium shows 2 distinct layers, i.e., outer chitinous and inner cellulose layer. A zonal pattern of sporangiospores development is uniquely characteristic of this pathogen: small, young spores are seen peripherally along the inner wall or form a crescent-like mass at one pole of the sporangium; medium-size, enlarging spores are between the periphery and at the center; and the larger, mature spores are centrally located. Mature sporangiospores appear lobulated due to globular eosinophilic inclusions and, when released into the tissue, can be suggestive of Prototheca. After development, it contains approximately 12,000–16,000 endospores. Size may increase by more than 450 μm. Ruptures of sprangium release endospores one by one via germinal pore.

Endospores—Enter surrounding connective tissue and develop into trophic stages. It is thought to be the asexual propagules of R. Seeberi. There is no evidence of a sexual stage in the life cycle of R. Seeberi. Mature endospores are spherical, measuring approximately 10–12 μm in diameter. It has a thick wall that is PAS positive, contains chitin. Several spherical bodies of approximately 1–1.5 μm in diameter; Vanbreuseghem et al. (1973) described endospores in Indian rhinosporidial tissue to be larger than those in African tissue [8].

The lamellated multilamellar body—Several authors have described these bodies as consisting of concentric rings of electron-dense material around a core of chromatin, and seen in juvenile and intermediate sporangia in human and animal rhinosporidial tissues.

Laminated body is stated as the precursors of the endospores in the study. Thianprasit et al. (1989) [13] and Apple et al. observed mature endospores and suggested that, after discharge from the sporangia, the endospores released the LB and from these arose the juvenile sporangia in continuation of the life cycle [14].

The life cycle of this organism in the tissues has two distinct phases:

1. Trophic.
2. Endosporulating, the diagnosis of rhinosporidiosis is based on detection of the cyst-like structures in the affected tissues [15].

The formation of the cyst wall appears to be a continuous morphological and biochemical spectrum throughout the cytological maturation of the organism; variations in this pattern have been noted to occur, probably as a protective mechanism, in concurrent rhinosporidiosis (Fig. 3.1 and Table 3.2) [1].

Mode of transmission—It is not definitely known. Moses et al. stated and supposed to be due to frequent exposure to water contaminated with spores of *Rhinosporidium seeberi* [16]. Jimenezet et al. opined that Conjunctival rhinosporidiosis is due to the infection that may arise by accidental eye injury by soil dust having the spores [17].

But the cultivation of organisms is not possible from the source to date. Reports of no detection of organisms after microscopic examination of deposits of stagnant water, silt, manure, and water plants in endemic areas have been confirmed the hypothesis of the aquatic habitat of R. seeberi. Deposits from ground waters in which rhinosporidiosis patients had taken bath had been processed to induce rhinosporidiosis in aquatic animals such as fish, snails, crabs, and frogs have also failed.

Fredricks et al. proposed that the natural hosts of R. seeberi are aquatic animals and mammalian hosts acquire infection via contaminated water. He also concluded that rhinosporidiosis is associated with exposure to water and aquatic parasites, but is also concluded that still there is a need for investigation of the infection in fish in ponds and rivers besides mammalian animals as reservoirs in disease endemic areas as well as screening antiparasitic drugs using infected fish or infected cell lines with nearest phylogenetic relatives of R. seeberi in DRIPs clade [3].

Ecology and Possible Sources

Epidemiological studies suggest that the main natural habitat of R. seeberi is groundwater in ponds and lakes, or in soil that is contaminated with such water. The evidences for it are mentioned in the studies include: a history given by the majority of Asian patients of exposure to these sources Studies by Noronha et al. (1933) [18] and of Mandlik et al. (1937) [19] observed that rhinosporidiosis of the nose [20] was closely associated with the occupation of sand-gathering from riverbeds. The outbreaks of rhinosporidiosis in humans were reported who had bathed in the common lake and in swans inhabiting the common lake [21, 22]. The higher prevalence in human males, through occupational exposure to soils and soil dust, a history of trauma from grass or wood splinters, sometimes related to agricultural occupations [21]. The occurrence of rhinosporidiosis in animals with an aquatic habitat, such as river dolphins, geese, swans, and ducks has been reported. The high frequency of

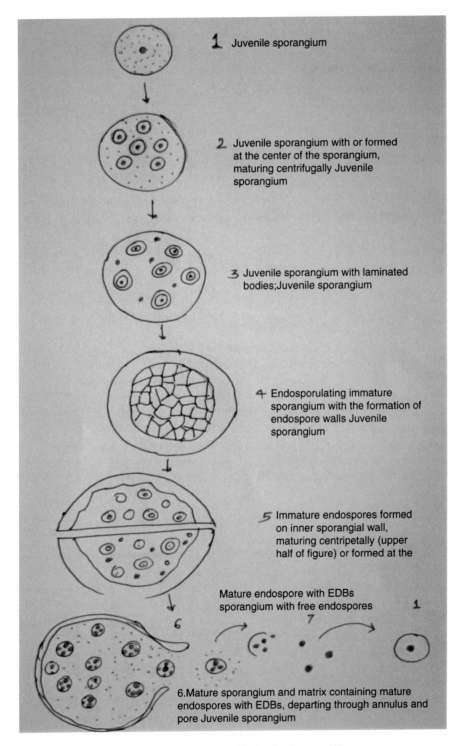

1 Juvenile sporangium

2 Juvenile sporangium with or formed at the center of the sporangium, maturing centrifugally Juvenile sporangium

3 Juvenile sporangium with laminated bodies;Juvenile sporangium

4 Endosporulating immature sporangium with the formation of endospore walls Juvenile sporangium

5 Immature endospores formed on inner sporangial wall, maturing centripetally (upper half of figure) or formed at the

Mature endospore with EDBs sporangium with free endospores

7

6.Mature sporangium and matrix containing mature endospores with EDBs, departing through annulus and pore Juvenile sporangium

Fig. 3.1 Various forms of Sporangia are observed in the development [2]

Table 3.2 Morphological features of sporangia of Rhinosporidium [2]

Characteristics	Juvenile sporangium	Intermediate sporangium	Mature sporangium
Size	6–10 μm in diameter	100–150 μm in diameter	100–450 μm in diameter
Morphology	Unilamellar,	Bilamellar wall, inner	Thinner bilamellar outer wall
Stain reaction		cellulose,	
PAS stain	Positive		Inner wall PAS-Mucicarmine-positive, variable
Mucicarmine	Negative	Positive	Outer wall PAS-, mucicarmine-and GMS-negative
GMS stain	GMS-negative wall Fibrillar or	Positive	Immature and mature
	granular,	Outer wall PAS-,	endospores present, embedded in matrix
	PAS-positive, mucicarmine	mucicarmine-and GMS-	Mature endospores with lipid
	GMS-negative cytoplasm	negative	globules and electron-dense
	Chromatin present as a single	No organized nucleus, lipid	bodies
	nucleus or as multiple nuclei,	globules present	
	each within a vesicle	Mature endospores absent	
	Laminated bodies present		
	Lipid globules present		

(PAS-Periodic acid–Schiff, GMS, Gomori's methenamine **silver**)

anterior urethral rhinosporidiosis in males was attributed to infection transported by pieces of stone or brick, probably contaminated by soilborne *R. seeberi*, applied to absorb the last drops of urine [23–25].

Kaluarachchi et al. (2008) developed the R. seeberi-specific fluorescein isothiocyanate (FITC)-labelled probe, and a complement of the R. seeberi-specific probe as a control probe, to investigate the groundwater habitat of R. seeberi by in situ hybridization and first time demonstrated the aquatic habitat of R. seeberi [20].

Entities were identified morphologically compatible structures with endospores and juvenile sporangia of R. seeberi. Spicules of sand particles in this water deposit were identified as a possible source of injury to the ocular and nasal mucosae that could initiate colonization by the aquatic R. seeberi. This is claimed as a first specific demonstration of the aquatic habitat of Rhinosporidium seeberi [2].

Cultivation of the Fungus

Culture on inanimate media—No attempt was proved to be successful to show the evidence of serial propagation, i.e., the repetition of the cycle of development of each stage to the mature sporangium, the release of its endospores and the repetition of the cycle of R. seeberi, on inanimate culture media.

When Grover (1970) suspended material from human rhinosporidial tissues in the synthetic medium TC 199 at 4 °C and observed a rapid increase in the number of endospores and the formation of sporangia; the organism was maintained for 4 months [26]. Arseculeratne et al. 1996 have made similar observations with Percoll-purified endospores (unpublished data) in phosphate-buffered saline or in tissue culture media, although the development did not proceed beyond the stage of immature sporangia; at no stage did we observe endosporulation in, and endo-sporerelease from, these sporangia [27].

Checking viability of organisms—Use of Nigrosin-eosin or Nigrosin-neutral red was found beneficial in the detection of viability through non-uptake of the dye [28]. Authors also used Evan's blue in a simple test for the assessment of the morphological integrity of R. seeberi's endospores; it is based on their staining by endospores were also found to stain deeply purple-blue with MTT which is used to assess the viability and hence the proliferation of lymphocytes in lymphoproliferative assays for cell-mediated immune competence, and for assessing the viability of fungi [29].

When Endospores were made inviable after autoclaving, formalization, and trypsinization, it failed to take up the Evan's blue or MTT, while endospores from freshly homogenized human rhinosporidial tissue stained deeply, in its cytoplasm and EDBs. Purified endospores after prolonged storage at −20 °C retained their staining with Evan's blue but failed to stain with MTT.

Staining with Evan's blue reveals the morphological integrity of the endospores, especially the EDBs, while MTT staining indicates their viability on account of the need for enzymic mechanisms (mitochondrial in eukaryotic cells) to reduce the MTT to the purple-blue colored formazan [29].

No tissue culture method after trying with incubation period at various temperatures proved successful for reproducible ontogenic development are as yet doubtful.

Attempts to Culture on Cell Lines

Levy et al. (1986) [30] and Easley et al. (1986) [31] tried the organism to grow the canine nasal rhinosporidiosis in monolayers of a cell line from an epithelioid human rectal tumor (HRT); Levy et al. observed the strong adherence of the organism within minutes to the cells and observed the polyp-like structures and mature sporangia releasing endospores into the medium after two days consisting of HRT cells. But there was no contest in polyps in cell cultures, which appeared within 2 days, and the polyps in clinical cases appear doubtful, not only in respect of the time interval of several months required for the development of the natural lesions, but also because the clinical polyps are consequent to the host's tissue response (epithelial proliferation, edema, with cellular infiltration into the fibrovascular stroma) surrounding the multiple sporangia and endospores. Easley et al. observed proliferation of the tumor cells around the organism, the numbers of which increased; the authors claimed that this reproduction' continued for over 3 months in subculture. No independent confirmation of these results has been reported [31].

Grover et al. reported the development of endospores into sporangia, and it was noted by Levy et al. (1986) who added that the development occurred also in the absence of the HRT cells [26, 30]. Arseculeratne et al. had observed the development of immature sporangia from endospores in HEp-2 or HeLa cells in MEM with 10 percent fetal calf serum, or even in phosphate buffered saline (PBS) pH 7.2

thawed after storage at $-20°C$ but not the formation of mature sporangia with mature endospores. Kennedy et al. not observed the growth of *R. seeberi* in fresh rhinosporidial tissue, in culture media with 10 percent fetal bovine serum [12].

- **Differential Histopathological Diagnosis.**

Infective diseases include rhinoscleroma, cryptococcosis, chromo(blasto) mycosis, histoplasmosis, infections caused by Chrysosporium (Emmonsia) parvum vars. parvum and crescens, blastomycosis, and paracoccidiodomycosis. Despite the ease of histopathological diagnosis through the ubiquitous developmental stages of R. seeberi in most rhizopodial tissue,

there are, however, problematic instances from which arise confusion, misdiagnosis, or a false-negative diagnosis. Arseculeratne et al. (2001) [32] mentioned these instances are when rhinosporidial bodies were absent in the rhinosporidial tissue despite the presence of marked cell infiltrates while other, more vascular, portions of the polyp, however, had rhinosporidial bodies; and justified that the problem occurs especially in the variegated polyps of nasopharyngeal rhinosporidiosis. Appropriate selection of portions of such polyps for histology might minimize the occurrence of a false-negative diagnosis (Table 3.3) [32].

Table 3.3 Morphological features of fungi showing spherule or likely structures in tissue [33]

Features	Rhinosporidium seeberi	Coccidioides immitis	Emmonsia crescens	Prototheca wickerhamii
Taxonomic status	Protista	Fungus	Fungus	Protista
Suze of spherules(μm)	10 – 450	60-100	50-500	7-13
Thickness of spherule walls	3-5	1-2	10-70	-
Size of endospores	6-10	2-5	-	2-11
Max. no. of endospores	16,000	200-300	-	50
Arthroconidia/Hyphae	_	Present	-	-
Pathological Reaction of Host	Acute/Chronic Inflammatory	Necrotic Granuloma	Fibrotic Granuloma	Necrotizing epitheloid Granuloma
Growth on Artificial Media	Non cultivable	Mycelial	Mycelial	Yeast like
Mucicarmine stain	Positive	Negative	Negative	Negative
GMS stain	Positive			
PAS stain	Positive			

Immunity

Antirhinosporidial antibody was not detected in patients by immunodiffusion or CIE by using suspensions of endospores and sporangia in a study by Chitravel et al. (1982) [34] and inferred that antigen preparations had insufficient amounts of soluble antigen. But Arseculeratne et al. performed CIE tests with antigens released by ultrasonic disintegration of Percoll-purified endospores/sporangia, and human rhinosporidial sera and detected precipitin lines [35].

Jayasekera et al. performed Rabbit experiments and Atapattu et al. in mice experiment detected Antirhinosporidial humoral immune responses (HIR) with indirect immunofluorescence tests by using Percoll-purified, sonically disrupted endospores and sporangia as antigen, respectively [36, 37].

Arseculeratne et al. (1999) detected IgG and IgM in patients' sera in immunodot blot assays on nitrocellulose paper, with specific antihuman immunoglobulin phosphatase conjugated tracers [38].

Cell-mediated immune (CMI) responses—Herr et al. (1999) [10] explained the various mechanisms of evasion of immune responses possibly chronicity, recurrence, and dissemination: antigenic variation. Immune suppression is demonstrated by de Silva et al. (2001) [4].

Immune distraction—Arseculeratne et al. reported cell infiltration to occur in some areas of the rhinosporidial tissue where rhinosporidial bodies are absent, suggesting that the infiltrates were due to reaction to free rhinosporidial antigen. In such cases, the possibility of immune distraction by free antigen might escape by antirhinosporidial antibody [32].

Cell-mediated immune responses (CMIR)—Human rhinosporidiosis were described by de Silva et al. The views put up were: immunohistochemistry with monoclonal antibodies against specific markers on cells in human rhinosporidial tissues and in vitro lymphoproliferative responses (LPR) of peripheral blood lymphocytes from rhinosporidial patients to the T-cell mitogen concanavalin A (conA) and to sonic extracts from Percoll-purified rhinosporidial endospores and sporangia.

The cell infiltrates in human rhinosporidial polyps showed uniformity in their origin from different clinical presentations with different durations. The composition of the cell infiltrate in human rhinosporidial polyps the infiltrates were mixed; neutrophils were abundant, CD20+ B cells were present in significant numbers with plasma cells, CD68+ macro- CD3+ T lymphocytes, were numerous. CD4+ helper T lymphocytes were scarce, while the presence of CD8+ T-cytotoxic/suppressor lymphocytes was marked; CD8 + cytotoxic/suppressor T lymphocytes were found specially around and within mature sporangia [38].

There were many TIA1-positive lymphocytes of the cytotoxic subtype located especially around the sporangia. CD56/57+ NK lymphocytes were less numerous than CD8+ T lymphocytes and were also located around mature sporangia [38].

In LPR assays in vitro (de Silva et al. 2001), demonstrate that while on the one hand a CMIR does develop in human rhinosporidiosis as well as suppressor responses also occur. In few patients, the peripheral blood lymphocytes showed a significantly lower proliferative response to rhinosporidial antigen than to conA, suggesting that the suppression was antigen-specific; the rhinosporidial antigen did not suppress the response to conA when the two agents were mixed, nor was the antigen toxic to the lymphocytes [38].

Immune deviation: Jayasekera et al. 2001 reported in the experimental studies on CMIR in mice to R. seeberi that occurrence of immune deviation might further contribute to immune evasion with decreasing antirhinosporidial CMI reactivity though antirhinosporidial CMIR is protective. Binding of host immunoglobulins [36].

Antigen sequestration: Abbas et al. reported that endospores have thick wall with chitin and cellulose and is possibly impermeable to release of antigens or to immune destruction of the endospores [39].

Grover et al. (1970) [26] reported the development of endospores into sporangia, and it was also noted by Levy et al. (1986) [30], who added that the development occurred also in the absence of the HRT cells. Arseculeratne et al. had observed the development of immature sporangia from endospores in HEp-2 or HeLa cells in MEM with 10 percent fetal calf serum, or even in phosphate buffered saline (PBS) pH 7.2 thawed after storage at $-20°C$ but not the formation of mature sporangia with mature endospores [27]. Kennedy et al. (1995) [12], not observed the growth of R. seeberi in fresh rhinosporidial tissue, in culture media with 10 percent fetal bovine serum.

- **Other Biological Activities.**

Hemagglutination—Arseculeratne and Atapattu et al. studied the Percoll-purified suspensions of endospores from human rhinosporidial tissues were found to cause hemagglutination of red blood cells from humans and rats. The hemagglutination occurred at 37 °C and at 4 °C [29].

Adherence-Endospores were reported to show strong adherence to epithelioid cells from a human rectal tumor, in vitro, HEp-2 cells in culture in Minimum Essential Medium (MEM) with calf serum [29].

Detection—Diagnosis depends on direct examination of infected tissue. GMS and PAS Stain -The walls of the sporangiospores and the mature sporangia are GMS and PAS positive.

Mucicarmine stain also will stain the walls of the spores and the inner surface of the sporangial wall. When periodic acid–Schiff (PAS) stained smears which are made from deposits of water from a reservoir in Sri Lanka in which many rhinosporidial patients had bathed were observed structures compatible in size and shape with rhinosporidial endospores and the presence within these bodies of structures that were also compatible with the electron-dense bodies (EDBs). Indirect immunofluorescence test with antirhinosporidial antibody showed extensive nonspecific labeling of amorphous, possibly mineral deposits in the water, which made identification of specifically labeled rhinosporidial bodies difficult [2].

Molecular studies on Rhinospodiosis on various aspects have been conducted:

- Vilela R the finding of synchronized nuclear division with the formation of endoconidia only in the latest mature stages, supports the placement of this unique pathogen in the mesomycetozoa and away from the fungi [40].
- Herr et al. [10] and Fredericks et al. [3] reported that the region of 18S SSU rRNA gene sequences of *R. seeberi* in human and other mammals with rhinosporidiosis were almost identical. Rhinosporidium was considered likely as a monotypic genus. But Silva et al. concluded in their study based on the complete internal transcribed spacer 1(ITS1), 5.8S, and ITS2 sequences of eight humans, two swans, and a dog with rhinosporidiosis and reported that the genus *Rhinosporidium* may possess multiple host-specific strains.

- **Sensitivity of *R. seeberi* to antimicrobial drugs.**

Conventional tests to antimicrobial drugs will not work due to inability to cultivate it. Researchers have tested many components, Quinine hydrochloride, salts of antimony and bismuth, iodine, and pentamidine griseofulvin, amphotericin B, and topical steroids local and systemic antibacterial antibiotics and radiotherapy but all proved to be ineffective clinically [17, 41–43].

An agent that is now used in therapy is dapsone (4,4'-diaminodiphenyl sulfone, DDS), and the evidence for its efficacy was obtained from clinical observations and microscopic examination of the pathogen in rhinosporidial tissue from treated patients.

The effects of antiseptics and disinfectants on the endospores of *Rhinosporidium seeberi was studied by* Arseculeratne et al. By using Evan's Blue (EvB), the integrity of morphological structures of the endospores was tested while with MTT (3-[4, 5-dimethylthiazol-2yl]-2, 5-diphenyl tetrazolium bromide) metabolic activity was detected through its reduction by cellular dehydrogenases to formazan which is insoluble microscopic deposits. Various disinfectants, i.e., hydrogen peroxide, glutaraldehyde, chloroxylenol, chlorhexidine, cetrimide, thimerosal, 70% ethanol, iodine in 70% ethanol, 10% formalin, povidone-iodine, sodium azide, and silver nitrate were tested on freshly harvested endospores. The disinfectants caused metabolic inactivation with or without disturbing the structural integrity as shown by the absence of MTT-staining after a contact time of 3, 24, or 36 hours [29].

Disinfectants like sodium azide, ethanol, thimerosal, chloroxylenol, glutaraldehyde, and hydrogen peroxide treated endospores are stained with EvB. Metabolic inactivation of the endospores was observed with a contact time of seven minutes with clinically useful biocides—chlorhexidine, cetrimide-chlorhexidine, 70% ethanol, povidone-iodine, and silver nitrate. Antiseptics that could be helpful in surgery on rhinosporidial patients include povidone-iodine in nasal packs for nasal and nasopharyngeal surgery, chlorhexidine, and cetrimide-chlorhexidine on the skin, while povidone-iodine and silver nitrate could have effective in ocular rhinosporidiosis [44].

An Area of Future Research

- Human leukocyte antigen type of the people in the endemic areas may be different when compared to the others.
- Biodiversity of the ponds that are different in the endemic regions.
- Physiochemical characteristics of water in India and Sri Lanka are more in favor of fungal growth when compared to the West.
- It is seen that incidence of rhinosporidiosis is more common in "O" blood group individuals (about 70%). What may be the cause?

References

1. Das S, Kashyap B, Barua M, Gupta N, Saha R, Vaid L, Banka A. Nasal rhinosporidiosis in humans: new interpretations and a review of the literature of this enigmatic disease. Med Mycol. 2011 Apr;49(3):311–315. https://doi.org/10.3109/13693786.2010.526640. Epub 2010 Oct 18.
2. Topley and Wilson's Microbiology and Microbial Infections, 8 Volume Set—AbeBooks—Topley, W. W. C.; Wilson: 0470686383 [Internet]. [cited 2021 Jul 31]. Available from: https://www.abebooks.com/9780470686386/Topley-Wilsons-Microbiology-Microbial-Infections-0470686383/plp.
3. Fredricks DN, Jolley JA, Lepp PW, Kosek JC, Relman DA. Rhinosporidium seeberi: a human pathogen from a novel group of aquatic protistan parasites. Emerg Infect Dis. 2000 May–Jun;6(3):273–82. https://doi.org/10.3201/eid0603.000307.
4. Silva V, Pereira CN, Ajello L, Mendoza L. Molecular evidence for multiple host-specifi c strains in the genus *Rhinosporidium*. J Clin Microbiol. 2005;43:1865–8.
5. Seeber GR. Un neuvo esporozuario parasito del hombre. Doscasos encontrades en polops nasales. Thesis, Fac Med Univ Nat de Buenos Aires; 1900.
6. Ciferri R, Redaelli P, Scatizzi I. Unita etiologica della melattia di Seeber (granuloma da Rhinosporidium seeberi) accertata con lo studio di materiali originali. Boll Soc Med Chir Pavia. 1936;14:723–45.
7. Ashworth JH. On Rhinosporidium seeberi (Wernicke 1903) with special reference to its sporulation and affinities. Trans R Soc Edinburg. 1923;53:301–42.
8. Vanbreuseghem R. Ultrastructure of Rhinosporidium seeberi. Int J Dermatol. 1973;12:20–8.
9. Ahluwalia KB, Maheswari N, et al. Rhinosporidiosis: a study that resolves etiologic controversies. Am J Rhinol. 1997;11(6):479–83.
10. Herr RA, Ajello L, Taylor JW, Arseculeratne SN, Mendoza L. Phylogenetic analysis of Rhinosporidium seeberi's 18S small-subunit ribosomal DNA groups this pathogen among members of the protoctistan Mesomycetozoa clade. J Clin Microbiol. 1999 Sep;37(9):2750–4.
11. Mendoza L, Taylor JW, Ajello L. The class mesomycetozoea: a heterogeneous group of microorganisms at the animal-fungal boundary. Annu Rev Microbiol. 2002;56:315–44.
12. Kennedy FA, Buggage RR, et al. Rhinosporidiosis: a description of an unprecedented outbreak in captive swans (Cygnus spp.) and a proposal for revision of the ontogenic nomenclature of Rhinosporidium seeberi. J Med Vet Mycol. 1995;37:157–65.
13. Thianprasit M, Thagernpol K. Rhinosporidiosis. Curr topics med Mycol, 3, 64–85 Savino, D.F. and Margo, C.E. 1983. Conjunctival rhinosporidiosis: light and electron microscopic study. Ophthalmology. 1989;99:1482–9.
14. Apple DJ. 'Papillome' der Conjunktiva bedingt durch Rhinosporidiose. Fortschr Ophthalmol. 1983;79:571–4.

15. Savino DF, Margo CE. Conjunctival rhinosporidiosis: light and electron microscopic study. Ophthalmology. 1983;99:1482–9.
16. Moses JS, Balachandran C, et al. Rhinosporidium seeberi: light, phase contrast, fluorescent and scanning electron microscopic study. Mycopathologia. 1991;114:17–20.
17. Jimenez JF, Young DE, et al. Rhinosporidiosis. A report of two cases from Arkansas. Am J Clin Pathol. 1984;82:611–5.
18. Noronha AJ. A preliminary note on the prevalence of rhinosporidiosis among sand-workers in Poona, with a brief description of some histological features of the rhinosporidial polypus. J Trop Med Hyg. 1933;36:115–20.
19. Mandlik GS. A record of rhinosporidial polypi with some observations on the mode of infection. Indian Med Gaz. 1937;72:143–7.
20. Kaluarachchi K, Sumathipala S, Eriyagama N, Atapattu D. The identification of the natural habitat of *Rhinosporidium seeberi* with *R. seeberi*-specific in situ hybridization probes. J Infect Dis Antimicrob Agents. 2008;25:25–32.
21. Karunaratne WAE. Rhinosporidiosis in man. London: The Athlone Press; 1964.
22. Vukovic Z, Bobic-Radovanovic A, et al. An epidemiological investigation of the first outbreak of rhinosporidiosis in Europe. J Trop Med Hyg. 1995;98:333–7.
23. Ingram AC. Rhinosporidium kinealyi in unusual situations. Lancet. 1910;2:726.
24. Dhayagude RG. Unusual rhinosporidial infection in man. Indian Med Gaz. 1941;76:513–5.
25. Gahukamble LD, John F, et al. Rhinosporidiosis of urethra. Trop Geog Med. 1982;34:266.
26. Grover R. Rhinosporidium seeberi: a preliminary study of the morphology and life cycle. Sabouraudia. 1970;7:249–51.
27. Arseculeratne SN, Mendoza L. Rhinosporidiosis. In: Merz WG, Hay RJ, editors. Topley & Wilson's microbiology and microbial infections, Vol. 4 32 J INFECT DIS ANTIMICROB AGENTS *Jan.-April 2008* medical mycology. 10th ed. London: Hodder Arnold; 2005. p. 436–5.
28. Jain SN. Aetiology and incidence of rhinosporidiosis. A preliminary report. Indian J Otolaryngol. 1967;19:1–21.
29. Arseculeratne SN, Atapattu DN Biological activities of the endospores of Rhinosporidium seeberi. Proc 25th Anniv Sessions, Kandy Soc Med, 23; 2003b.
30. Levy MG, Meuten DJ, et al. Cultivation of Rhinosporidium seeberi in vitro: interaction with epithelial cells. Science. 1986;234:474–6.
31. Easley JR, Meuten DJ, et al. Nasal rhinosporidiosis in the dog. Vet Pathol. 1986;23:50–6.
32. Arseculeratne SN, Panabokke RG, et al. Lymphadenitis, transepidermal elimination and unusual histopathology in human rhinosporidiosis. Mycopathologia. 2001;153:57–69.
33. de Hoog GS, Guarro J, Gené J, Ahmed S, Al-Hatmi AMS, Figueras MJ, Vitale RG. Atlas of clinical fungi. 4th ed. Hilversum; 2020.
34. Chitravel V, Sundararaj V, et al. Cell mediated immune response in human cases of rhinosporidiosis. Sabouraudia. 1981;19:135–42.
35. Arseculeratne SN, Atapattu DN, et al. The humoral immune response in human rhinosporidiosis. Proc Kandy Soc Med. 1999;21:19.
36. Jayasekera S, Arseculeratne SN, et al. Cell-mediated immune responses (CMIR) to Rhinosporidium seeberi in mice. Mycopathologia. 2001;152:69–79.
37. Atapattu DN, Arseculeratne SN, et al. Purification of the endospores and sporangia of Rhinosporidium seeberi on Percoll columns. Mycopathologia. 1999;145:113–9.
38. de Silva NR, Huegel H, et al. Cell-mediated immune responses (CMIR) in human rhinosporidiosis. Mycopathologia. 2001;152:59–68.
39. Abbas AK, Lichtman AH, Pober JS. Cellular and molecular immunology. Philadelphia: W.B. Saunders; 2000. p. 359.
40. Vilela R, Mendoza L. The taxonomy and phylogenetics of the human and animal pathogen Rhinosporidium seeberi: a critical review. Rev Iberoam Micol. 2012 Oct–Dec;29(4):185–199. https://doi.org/10.1016/j.riam.2012.03.012. Epub 2012 Apr 12.

41. Rajam RV, Viswanathan GC, et al. Rhinosporidiosis: a study with a report of a fatal case with systemic dissemination. Indian J Surg. 1955;17:269–98.
42. Ho MS, Tay BK. Disseminated rhinosporidiosis. Ann Acad Med Singap. 1986;15:80–3.
43. Satyanarayana C. Rhinosporidiosis. In: Elbs M, editor. Clinical surgery. London: Butterworth; 1966. p. 143–52.
44. Arseculeratnes SN, Atapattu DN, Balasooriya P, Fernando R. The effects of biocides (antiseptics and disinfectants) on the endospores of Rhinosporidium seeberi. Indian J Med Microbiol. 2006;24(2):85–91.

Clinical Presentation: ENT Spectrum

Rupa Mehta, Nidhin SB, and Nitin M. Nagarkar

Rhinosporidiosis is a distinctive granulomatous infection of the mucocutaneous region. It has been known since long; the disease is endemic in certain states of India such as Chhattisgarh, Tamil Nadu, Kerala, Orissa, and eastern Madhya Pradesh [1]. Our institute being one of the major referral centers in central India has a vast experience in diagnosing and managing variety of typical and atypical rhinosporidiosis. Here in this chapter, we will be discussing our experience of managing 152 otolaryngological rhinosporidiosis cases over last 3 years.

Out of total 152 histological proven operated cases of rhinosporidiosis, there were 108 (71%) males and 44 (28%) females. In literature, the ratio of male to female incidence of this disease varies from 1.3:1 to 9:1.9. A few studies have shown female predominance also. The reason for the lower number of females affected might be less frequent pond baths [2]. Some authors are of the opinion that estrogen may have a protective role [3]. In our experience mean age of presentation was 23 years with a range of 6 to 70 years. Sinha et al. [4] and Manonmany et al. [5] have found that 20 to 40 years were the most affected age group. In a study by Karthikeyan et al. [6], 21 to 50 years were the most commonly affected age group, with 31 to 40 years age group being even more predominant. Hence, we can conclude that mostly young and middle-aged persons are affected by rhinosporidiosis. In our experience majority of the patients were from rural area 127(84%) followed by semi-urban 15(10%) and urban 10(7%). We noted most of the patients were daily wage laborers followed by school going children belonging to low socioeconomic

R. Mehta (✉) · N. SB · N. M. Nagarkar
Department of ENT and Head Neck Surgery, AIIMS, Raipur, India

N. M. Nagarkar, R. Mehta (eds.), *Rhinosporidiosis*,
https://doi.org/10.1007/978-981-16-8508-8_4

status. All cases had history of bathing in ponds and lakes. In our study, O +ve blood group was seen in majority of patients, followed almost equally by AB +ve, B +ve, and A +ve. Kameswaran et al. [7] reported maximum incidence rate of rhinosporidiosis in blood group O (70%), followed by blood group AB. However, Jain et al. [8] denied the role of blood group as a predisposing factor for rhinosporidiosis.

In our experience otorhinolaryngological rhinosporidiosis can be divided into:

1. Nasal (109) 71.7%
2. Nasal + Nasopharyngeal (20) 13.1%
3. Nasal + Nasopharyngeal + Oropharyngeal (12) 7.8%
4. Laryngo - hypopharyngeal (4) 2.6%
5. Nasolacrimal duct (5) 3.2%
6. Parotid duct (2) 1.3%

In our study, 80% patients had unilateral involvement and 20% patient had bilateral presentation. Seventy-percent of patient had multifocal involvement, rest 30% had unifocal involvement. No predilection to any specific side of the nasal cavity was seen, both right and left sides were affected almost equally. Manonmony et al. [5], in their study, found a higher incidence on the right side of the nasal cavity (47%), followed by left side (33%). The most common symptom of rhinosporidiosis was nasal obstruction, followed by epistaxis, nasal discharge, and nasal mass. Similar findings have been found in other studies. In a study of nasal rhinosporidiosis cases by Guru and Pradhan et al. [9], the lateral wall of the nose, followed by the septum and floor, was the most common site of attachment of the mass. Karthikeyan et al. [6] found the septum, followed by the inferior turbinate and inferior meatus, as the most common site of attachment. In our study, the inferior turbinate and floor were the most common sites, followed by the nasal septum, lateral wall, and nasopharynx. Soft palatal involvement was also seen which usually causes stricture and fibrosis. In our case series, we had 4 cases of laryngeal, 3 cases of extensive oropharyngeal rhinosporidiosis, 1 patient had lesion over the tongue, soft palate, and post pharyngeal wall. In all these cases, we did tracheostomy and then proceeded for surgery. In many patients, especially with extensive oropharyngeal involvement, cystic and polypoidal changes were also seen in the oropharyngeal masses.

In all our cases we did thorough history taking, clinical examination, Diagnostic nasal endoscopy and Video laryngoscopy. CECT scan was done for patients presenting with extensive disease, recurrent disease, and oropharyngeal and laryngeal involvement. Endoscopic Excision of rhinosporidial mass was done for all cases.

For 4 cases of laryngohypopharyngeal rhinosporidiosis, we performed micro-laryngeal surgery with debulking. Bipolar cauterization of the base was done after complete excision for all cases to reduce the chances of recurrence. Microdebrider, and coblation were also used for excision of the lesions.

High chance of recurrence is seen in rhinosporidiosis even after complete surgery. According to the literature, recurrence rate ranges from 5 to 63% [7]. Thirty out of the 152 cases in the our study had (19.73%) recurrence. Vadakkan et al. [10], in their study, mentioned a case having 42 episodes of recurrent nasal and nasopharyngeal rhinosporidiosis. Similarly, in our study, 1 patient had 12 episodes of recurrent nasal and naso oropharyngeal rhinosporidiosis. 2 patients with disseminated rhinosporidiosis had 8–10 times recurrence. For all recurrent and disseminated rhinosporidiosis dapsone was started after excluding G6PD deficiency for 3 months with monitoring of haemoglobin (Figs. 4.1, 4.2, 4.3, 4.4, 4.5, 4.6, 4.7, 4.8, 4.9, 4.10, 4.11, 4.12, 4.13, 4.14 and 4.15).

Fig. 4.1 Total number of patients & male, female distribution

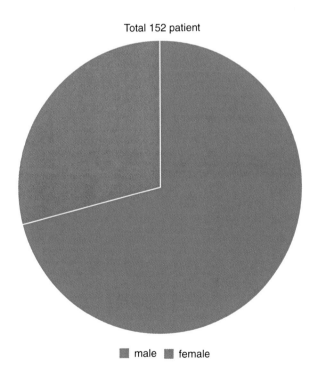

Total 152 patient

male ■ female

Fig. 4.2 Demography of
rhinosporidiosis patient

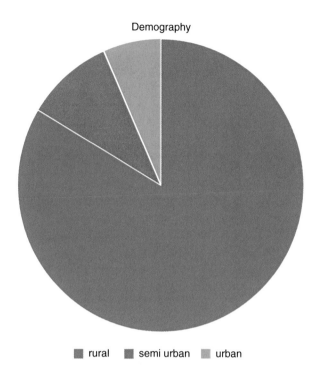

Demography

rural   semi urban   urban

Fig. 4.3 Blood group
distribution

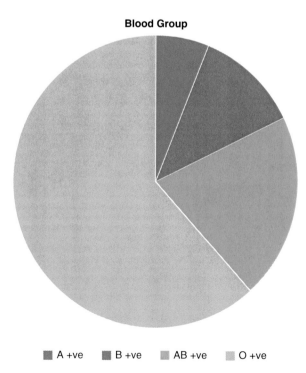

Blood Group

A +ve   B +ve   AB +ve   O +ve

Fig. 4.4 Laterality of
presentation

laterality of presentation

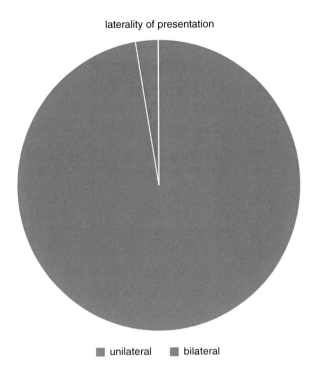

■ unilateral ■ bilateral

Fig. 4.5 Focality of lesion

focality of lesion

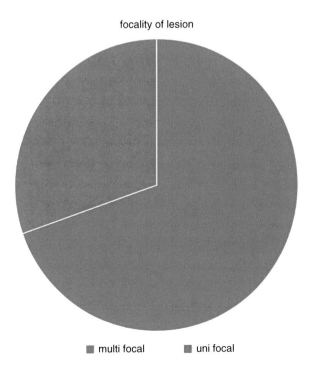

■ multi focal ■ uni focal

Fig. 4.6 Symptomatology

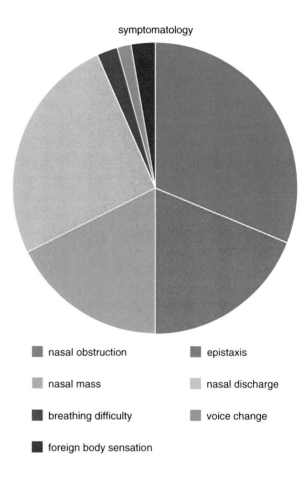

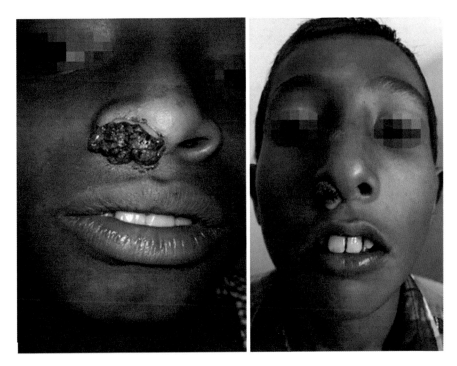

Fig. 4.7 Rhinosporidiosis mass arising out of right nasal cavity

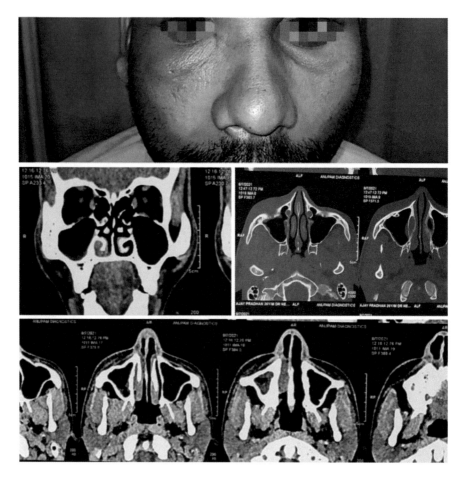

Fig. 4.8 Right side nasolacrimal duct rhinosporidiosis

Fig. 4.9 Pyriform
sinus and aryeepiglottic
fold rhinosporidiosis

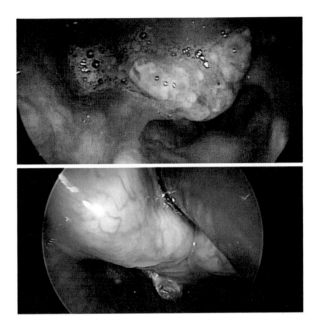

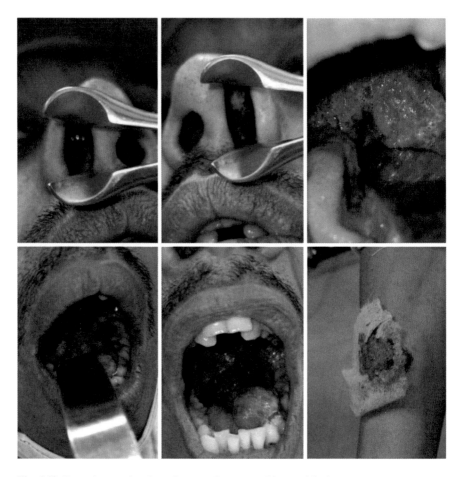

Fig. 4.10 Extensive nasal and oropharyngeal recurrent rhinosporidiosis

Fig. 4.11 Laryngeal
rhinosporidiosis

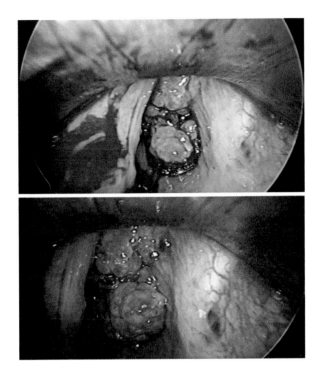

Fig. 4.12 Bilateral nasal
and nasopharyngeal
rhinsporidiosis

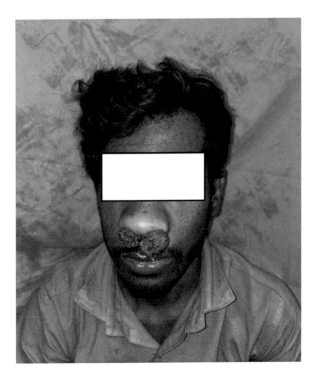

Fig. 4.13 Oropharyngeal rhinosporidiosis

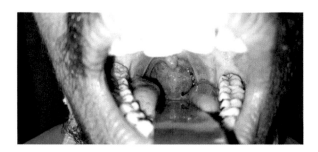

Fig. 4.14 Recurrent nasolacrimal rhinosporidiosis

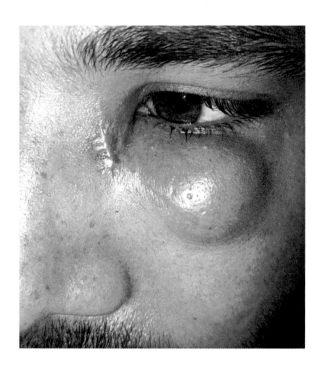

Fig. 4.15 Parotid duct
rhinosporidiosis

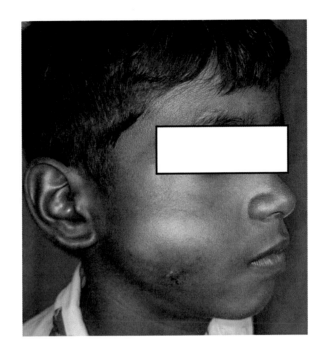

References

1. Ghorpade A. Giant cutaneous rhinosporidiosis. J Eur Acad Dermatol Venereol. 2006;20(01):88–9.
2. Herr RA, Mendoza L, Arseculeratne SN, Ajello L. Immunolocalization of an endogenous antigenic material of Rhinosporidium seeberi expressed only during mature sporangial development. FEMS Immunol Med Microbiol. 1999;23(03):205–12.
3. Jayasekera S, Arseculeratne SN, Atapattu DN, Kumarasiri R, Tilakaratne WM. Cell-mediated immune responses (CMIR) to Rhinosporidium seeberi in mice. Mycopathologia. 2001;152(02):69–79.
4. Sinha A, Phukan JP, Bandyopadhyay G, et al. Clinicopathological study of rhinosporidiosis with special reference to cytodiagnosis. J Cytol. 2012;29(04):246–9.
5. Manonmany S, Renjit RE, Philip JT, Raj AR. Rhinosporidiosis: analysis of cases presenting to a tertiary care hospital in rural Kerala. Int J Biomed Res. 2015;6:416–20.
6. Karthikeyan P, Vijayasundaram S, Pulimoottil DT. A retrospective epidemiological study of rhinosporidiosis in a rural tertiary care centre in Pondicherry. J Clin Diagn Res. 2016;10(5):MC04.
7. Kameswaran S, Lakshmanan M. Rhinosporidiosis. In: Kameswaran S, Kameswaran M, editors. ENT disorders in a tropical environment. Chennai: MERF Publications; 1999. p. 19–34.
8. Jain SN. Aetiology and incidence of rhinosporidiosis. Indian J Otolaryngol. 1967;19(1):1–21.
9. Guru RK, Pradhan DK. Rhinosporidiosis with special reference to extra nasal presentation. J Evol Med Dent Sci. 2014;3(22):6189–99. https://doi.org/10.14260/jemds/2014/2721.
10. Vadakkan JR, Ganeshbala A, Jalagandesh B. A clinical study of rhinosporidiosis in rural coastal population: our experience. J Evol Med Dent Sci. 2014;3(51):11938–42. https://doi.org/10.14260/jemds/2014/3575.

Clinical Presentation: Ophthalmological Spectrum

Somen Misra and Neeta Misra

Introduction

Rhinosporidiosis is a granulomatous disease caused by Rhinosporidium seeberi. It mainly affects anatomical locations lined by mucous membrane. Rhinosporidiosis inflict all the mucosa that open on the exterior [1]. Conjunctiva, nasal mucosa, and vaginal mucosa are the most commonly affected sites, anal mucosa being the most rarely affected location. Periocular lesion from mucosal extension has been reported. Intra-ocular manifestation has not been found. Ocular rhinosporidiosis most often presents as a polypoid mass of the palpebral conjunctiva [2]. It may also present as a lacrimal sac diverticulum, recurrent chalazion, conjunctival cyst, chronic follicular conjunctivitis, peripheral keratitis, scleral melting, ciliary staphyloma or simulate a tumour of eyelid or periorbital skin. It affects both adults and children. Men are affected more than women [3]. The diagnosis is confirmed by histopathology of the biopsied specimen. Definitive management is wide surgical excision with wide area electrocoagulation of the lesion base. Recurrences of ocular rhinosporidiosis have rarely been reported. Traumatic autoinoculation from one site to another by fingers is common [4].

Epidemiology

The disease has been reported from 70 tropical countries on either side of the equator. The disease is common in areas with high and prolonged rainfall. It is mainly prevalent in the Indian subcontinent, particularly in India and Sri Lanka, and in South American countries such as Argentina and Brazil. Most of the cases have

S. Misra (✉) · N. Misra
Department of Ophthalmology, AIIMS, Raipur, India

© The Author(s), under exclusive license to Springer Nature Singapore Pte Ltd. 2022
N. M. Nagarkar, R. Mehta (eds.), *Rhinosporidiosis*,
https://doi.org/10.1007/978-981-16-8508-8_5

47

been reported from India, Sri Lanka and Bangladesh. Cases reported from outside the Indian subcontinent are mostly amongst migrants from India. It has been shown that over 90% of patients are from Asia, while South America accounts for fewer than 5% of the total cases [5]. Despite its high endemicity in India, distribution throughout the country is not uniform. It is quite prevalent in Tamil Nadu, Kerala and other states of south India [6]. Cases have been rarely reported from states of Northern India like Punjab, Himachal Pradesh and Haryana [7, 8]. Chhattisgarh is an endemic region for rhinosporidiosis infection in Central India. This high prevalence can be explained by a suitable hot tropical environment as well as a social practice of common bathing of the public with animals outdoor, mainly in ponds and rivers. Sudarshan V et al. reported 462 cases during a period of 12 years from January 1994 to December 2005 in Raipur only [9].

Mode of Transmission

The commonest hypothesis is that the disease is waterborne and the disease condition passes from animal to man. The commonest mode is from infected water buffaloes to human beings sharing the same pond [10]. The exact mode of transmission is still not known. It has been hypothesized that direct transmission of the spores of the organism may happen on an exposed mucosal surface through dust, water or through infected clothing or fingers. Spread from human to human has not been established. All people living in the same house and bathing in the same pond do not develop the disease. It is uncommon for more than one person to be infected in the same family. The occurrence of autoinoculation is shown by the development of growth at newer sites nearby conjunctiva and lacrimal involvement.

Trauma might play an important role in the causation of the disease since there is no evidence that the spores can gain entrance through intact epithelium once they had been discharged outside the limiting epithelium of the mass [11] (Fig. 5.1).

Fig. 5.1 Animals and humans taking bath in the same pond

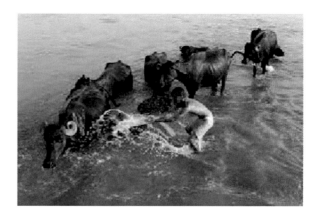

Classification

Till 1963, all periocular involvements were thought to be an extension from the nose. In 1963, Kuriacose divided it into primary rhinosporidiosis and secondary rhinosporidiosis [12].

Mukherjee PK (1980) divided Oculosporidiosis into Conjunctivosporidiosis and Dacryosporidiosis [13].

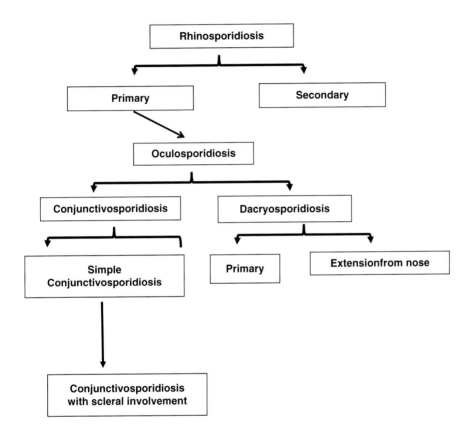

Signs of Conjunctivo Sporidiosis

It presents as a fleshy mass on visible part of the conjunctiva and fornices. The mass can be lifted from conjunctiva. If located at the fornices, it is usually found to be pedunculated. It is found as a sessile mass in both tarsal and Bulbar conjunctiva. It usually bleeds profusely during surgical manipulation. The mass appears like white semolina(sujee) granules on the surface [13].

Different Clinical Presentation of Conjunctivo Sporidiosis

Fig. 5.2 Left eye with bulbar lesion extending outside the conjunctival sac (Courtesy: Dr. P.K. Mukherjee)

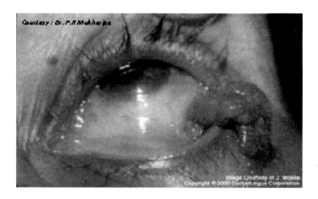

Fig. 5.3 Right eye upper tarsal lesion (Courtesy: Dr. P.K. Mukherjee)

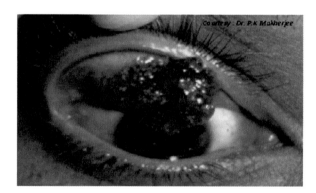

Fig. 5.4 Left eye with Upper fornix involvement (Courtesy: Dr. P.K. Mukherjee)

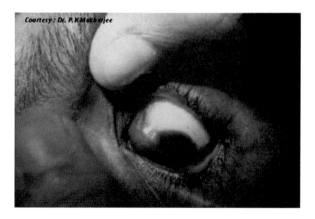

Fig. 5.5 Left eye with lower bulbar conjunctival involvement

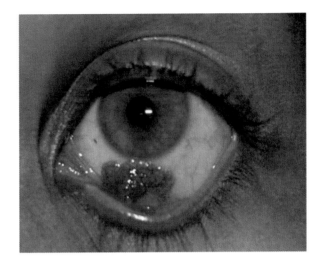

Fig. 5.6 Left eye with a lesion involving upper fornix and conjunctiva

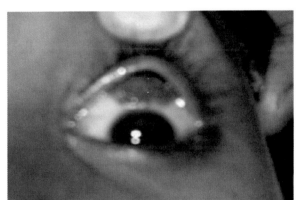

Fig. 5.7 Right eye pedunculated lesion involving upper eyelid margin

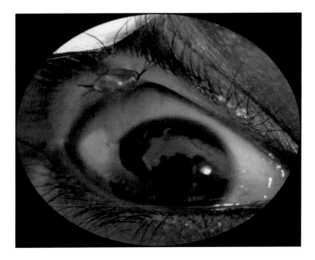

Clinical Presentation with Scleral Involvement
in Ocular Rhinosporidiosis

Fig. 5.8 Right eye with
supero-temporal scleral
lesion (Courtesy: Dr.
P.K. Mukherjee)

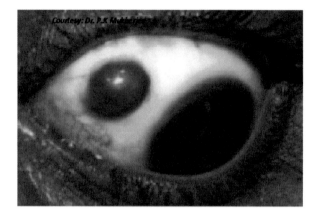

Fig. 5.9 Right eye with a
lesion at 12 o'clock
position straddling the
limbus (Courtesy: Dr.
P.K. Mukherjee)

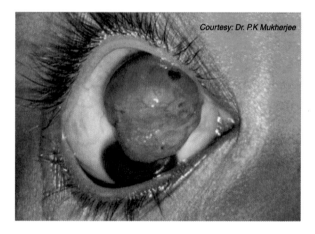

Investigation of Ocular Rhinosporidiosis

Microscopy

This is a simple clinical test in which a small piece of the lesion is removed under local anaesthesia. It is teased thin with a hypodermic needle, then a drop of normal saline is put. It is covered with a cover slide and microscopic examination is done under high power. Sporangia can be seen standing out prominently. The above examination can be done under 10% KOH that has the added advantage of dissolving the conjunctival tissue. Histopathology of excised mass can be done in which staining with haematoxylin and Eosin is done. Fine needle aspiration from the lacrimal sac and adjoining structure is routinely done. Regurgitated fluid from the sac is collected on slide, fixed and examined routinely [14].

Differential Diagnosis of Conjunctivo Sporidiosis

"All fleshy mass in the conjunctiva in endemic area should be considered to be rhinosporidiosis unless proven otherwise". Pathologies that can mimic conjunctivo sporidiosis are burst chalazion, infective granuloma and foreign body granuloma. Dysplastic conditions having similar presentations as rhinosporidiosis are papilloma and haemangioma which are benign lesions presenting in people of younger age group and epidermoid carcinoma which is a malignant condition seen in older individuals.

Treatment of Conjunctivo Sporidiosis

To date no medical treatment is available. Definitive treatment is surgical removal of the mass. It can be done routinely as an outdoor procedure or can be done as an elective case in an operation theatre set up under strict sterile measures. The stump is excised with the application of diathermy or cryo application. It bleeds profusely during surgical manipulation, care has to be taken to secure the bleeders with the help of cryoprobe or electrocautery. No recurrence has been reported when removed completely. It is surprising to know that no recurrence has been found afterwards even if the patient lives in the same environment.

Dacryocystosporidiosis

Lacrimal sac is the commonest site to be infected among all the periocular tissue involved in rhinosporidiosis. Infection of lacrimal gland has never been reported. It can be primary dacryocystosporidiosis, i.e. lacrimal sac involvement without involvement of nose. Extension from nose is less frequent. Unilateral involvement is more common. It is more common in children. It usually presents as a chronic painless and non-tender mass [13]. It has been found localized in the sac without involving pericystic tissue. If there is pericystic involvement, it results in a diffuse swelling that spreads from sac towards the lower lid. The skin over the growth is not fixed. The skin has an orange peel-like appearance. The swelling is not reducible and non-compressible. Temperature over the swelling is usually found normal [14].

Peculiarity of Lacrimal Passage in Dacryocystosporidiosis

There are few clinical presentations that help us in differentiating dacryocystosporidiosis from other lacrimal masses. In a patient with dacryocystosporidiosis, there is hardly any epiphora and no regurgitation of fluid on pressure over the lacrimal sac is seen. The canaliculi are found patent in most of the cases. On syringing, the nasolacrimal duct is found open or partially open. In case of the partially open nasolacrimal duct, the swelling increases in size when fluid is pushed and it takes some time for saline to reach the throat and on pressing the lacrimal sac saline regurgitates from the puncta. If saline is not forced out, the saline causes inflammatory reaction that leads to pericystitis that may cause cellulitis, abscess formation, formation of fistula, and protrusion of the lesion through the fistula. Dacryocystography with oil-based opaque substance causes severe pericystitis, so it is contraindicated and the radiopaque agent needs to be washed away with normal saline, once the procedure is done. Computed tomography of the sac, paranasal sinus and orbit is helpful in visualizing lesions with deeper tissue involvement.

Dacryosporidiosis Clinical Presentation

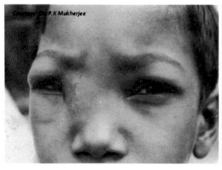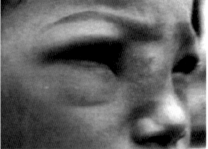

Figs. 5.10 and 5.11 Right nasolacrimal duct involvement causing swelling from medial canthus to midline in horizontal axis, brow to ala of nose in vertical axis

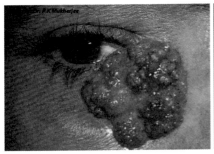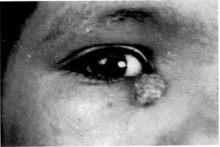

Figs. 5.12 and 5.13 Fungating lesion of dacryocystosporidiosis due to rupture of pericystic abscess

Causes of Lacrimal Fistula in Rhinosporidiosis

In untreated cases, rupture of pericystic abscess, incision of pericystic cellulitis, deliberate incision of the swelling may cause inadvertent lacrimal fistula.

Probable Route of Infection in Dacryocystosporidiosis

Retrograde inoculation from the nose, though relatively rare, but has been reported. Anterograde spread from conjunctivo sporidiosis has been commonly seen. In adults chronic dacryocystitis, i.e. pre-existing block in nasolacrimal duct can lead to stagnation of infective spores and further disease manifestation. Untreated and partially treated congenital nasolacrimal duct obstruction could be an inciting factor in paediatric age group. Children following exanthematous diseases like chickenpox, measles have been found presenting with dacryosporidiosis.

Treatment of Dacryocystosporidiosis

To date, no known medical treatment is available. Many trials have been conducted with drugs like dapsone and rifampicin but with no conclusive results. Surgery is the definitive treatment that is removal of the growth in toto. If a small bit of infected tissue is left, recurrence is unavoidable.

There are two routes for surgical excision—classical transcutaneous and endonasal route. Transnasal excision of the growth under direct vision. Once the sac is removed, conjunctivo rhinoanastomosis is a viable but difficult alternative to correct epiphora.

Unexplained Aspects of Rhinosporidiosis

There are many unexplained aspects of rhinosporidiosis. On the top of the list is the position of the organism in the world of microbiology, whether it is a fungus, a protozoa, an algae or something else? It has still not been cultured. It has not been produced experimentally in animals. Why lymph nodes are not involved? There is no recurrence following complete removal even if the patient lives in the same environment. There may be an immunological cause for non-recurrence. Only one person in the family gets the disease. Why conjunctival sporidiosis is not always associated with dacryocystosporidiosis? Corneal involvement is not known. No intraocular involvement has been reported, though scleral involvement is not rare. Why children are affected more? Why there is no effective medical treatment?

Conclusion

Rhinosporidiosis is a chronic granulomatous infection affecting mucous membranes caused by Rhinosporidium seeberi. It belongs to the class Protista classified under Mesomycetozoa. The disease is endemic in South India, Sri Lanka, South America and Africa. It is mainly transmitted by exposure to contaminated water. It can occur in two forms, i.e. conjunctivo sporidiosis and dacryocystosporidiosis. The diagnosis is confirmed by histopathology of the biopsied specimen. Definitive management is wide surgical excision with wide area electrocoagulation of the lesion base. Recurrences are very rare.

References

1. Chitravel V, Sundararaj T, Subramanian S, Kumaresan M, Kunjithapadam S. Cell mediated immune response in human cases of rhinosporidiosis. Sabouraudia. 1981;19(2):135–42.
2. Jain K, Dewan T, Paliwal P, Singh MD, Gupta S. Ocular Rhinosporidiosis presenting as a rapidly growing conjunctival papilloma. Off Sci J Delhi Ophthalmol Soc. 2018;28(3):32–4.
3. Ghosh AK, De Sarkar A, Bhaduri G, Datta A, Das A, Bandyopadhyay A. Ocular rhinosporidiosis. J Indian Med Assoc. 2004;102(12):732–64.
4. Varshney S, Bist S, Gupta P, Gupta N, Bhatia R. Lacrimal sac diverticulum due to Rhinosporidiosis. Indian J Otolaryngol Head Neck Surg. 2007;59(4):353–6.
5. Van der Coer J, Marres H, Wlelinga E, Wong-Alcala L. Rhinosporidiosis in Europe. J Laryngol Otol. 1992;106(5):440–3.
6. Moses J, Balachandran C. Rhinosporidiosis in bovines of Kanyakumari district, Tamil Nadu, India. Mycopathologia. 1987;100(1):23–6.
7. Moses J, Shanmugham A, Kingsly N, Vijayan J, Balachandran C, Albert A. Epidemiological survey of rhinosporidiosis in Kanyakumari district of Tamil Nadu. Mycopathologia. 1988;101(3):177–9.
8. Samaddar R, Sen M. Rhinosporidiosis in Bankura. Indian J Pathol Microbiol. 1990;33(2):129–36.

9. Sudarshan V, Goel N, Gahine R, Krishnani C. Rhinosporidiosis in Raipur, Chhattisgarh: a report of 462 cases. Indian J Pathol Microbiol. 2007;50(4):718–21.
10. Chitravel V, Sundaram B, Subramanian S, Kumaresan M, Kunjithapatham S. Rhinosporidiosis in man. Mycopathologia. 1990;109(1):11–2.
11. Gupta R, Darbari B, Dwivedi M, Billore O, Arora M. An epidemiological study of rhinosporidiosis in and around Raipur. Indian J Med Res. 1976;64(9):1293–9.
12. Kuriakose E. Oculosporidiosis: rhinosporidiosis of the eye. Br J Ophthalmol. 1963;47(6):346.
13. Mukherjee P, Jain P, Mishra R. Exanthemata: a causative factor of chronic dacryocystitis in children. Indian J Ophthalmol. 1969;17(1):27.
14. Nuruddin M, Mudhar HS, Osmani M, Roy SR. Lacrimal sac rhinosporidiosis: clinical profile and surgical management by modified dacryocystorhinostomy. Orbit. 2014;33(1):29–32.

Clinical Presentation: Dermatological Spectrum

Neel Prabha

Introduction

Cutaneous involvement in rhinosporidiosis is infrequent. Forsyth, in 1942 first described a case of cutaneous rhinosporidiosis secondary to nasal rhinosporidiosis [1]. Since then, few other cases of cutaneous rhinosporidiosis have been reported in the literature; most of them are from India. Ghorpade proposed the term dermosporidiosis for cutaneous involvement in rhinosporidiosis [2]. The incidence of cutaneous rhinosporidiosis ranges from 0.39 to 8.33% [3, 4].

Etiopathogenesis: *Rhinosporidium Seeberi*, the causative organism of rhinosporidiosis, commonly involves the upper respiratory tract and enters through the traumatized epithelium in nasal sites from the natural habitat [5]. Rarely skin is also involved. Various modes of infection/spread are described in cutaneous rhinosporidiosis. These are:

1. **Autoinoculation**: Autoinoculation of *Rhinosporidium Seeberi* spores is responsible for satellite lesions around the nose in a case of nasal rhinosporidiosis [6]. However, lesions at distant sites due to autoinoculation have also been described. Sirka et al. have described a case of nasal rhinosporidiosis who developed cutaneous lesions on the right little finger and left popliteal fossa possibly due to autoinoculation [7]. Nath et al. also described a case of nasopharyngeal rhinosporidiosis where nail involvement occurred by autoinoculation [8]. The infection spreads through abrasions on the adjacent or distant skin surface by autoinoculation of exogenous endospores present on the primary involved epithelial surface. The abrasions can be caused by scratching the skin with the infected fingernail (caused by nose fingering).

N. Prabha (✉)
Department of Dermatology, All India Institute of Medical Sciences, Raipur, India

© The Author(s), under exclusive license to Springer Nature Singapore Pte Ltd. 2022
N. M. Nagarkar, R. Mehta (eds.), *Rhinosporidiosis*,
https://doi.org/10.1007/978-981-16-8508-8_6

2. **Hematogenous spread**: This mode of spread is the most common cause of cutaneous rhinosporidiosis. Generalized skin involvement occurs due to hematogenous dissemination of infection after the *Rhinosporidium seebri* enters the blood circulation [9]. Generalized skin involvement with or without nasal involvement is seen.

3. **Lymphatic spread**: The role of lymphatics in spreading rhinosporidiosis is controversial. Arseculeratne et al. suggested that lymphatic spread can occur in rhinosporidiosis [10]. Arseculeratne et al. found rhinosporidial sporangia in an inguinal lymph node biopsy of a patient of disseminated rhinosporidiosis with lesions in the leg, confirming the role of lymphatic spread in rhinosporidiosis [10].

4. **Direct inoculation**: This mode of infection is uncommon. Primary cutaneous lesions develop by direct inoculation of the organism from the natural aquatic habitat into the skin.

In the case of cutaneous rhinosporidiosis, both autoinoculation and the hematogenous spread can be seen. The appearance of cutaneous lesions suggests the possibility of autoinoculation spread, while subcutaneous lesions with intact overlying skin suggest the possibility of hematogenous spread [11].

Clinical Features of Cutaneous Rhinosporidiosis

Based upon the modes of spread, three types of cutaneous lesions have been described. They are: [1] Satellite lesions, [2] Disseminated lesions, and [3] Primary cutaneous type.

1. **Satellite lesions**: Satellite lesions adjacent to granulomas occur due to autoinoculation. Satellite lesions are commonly seen in the skin adjacent to nasal mucosa due to contiguous spread from the nasal mucosa [12]. In this type of cutaneous rhinosporidiosis, visceral involvement is not seen.

2. **Disseminated lesions**. Hematogenous spread from the primary respiratory site is responsible for the development of lesions to anatomically distant sites. Disseminated lesions can appear as early as 4 months to as late as 26 years of primary infection [8, 12–19]. Occasionally, visceral lesions can also develop. The majority of cutaneous lesions are seen as a component of disseminated rhinosporidiosis. These lesions are generally present with mucosal lesions. However, due to the spread of infection from subclinical infection in the upper respiratory site, cutaneous lesions without mucosal lesions have also been reported [20]. Date et al. [20] described a case that presented with only a cutaneous lesion. When the diagnosis of cutaneous rhinosporidiosis was confirmed by biopsy, the nasopharynx was examined, and mucosa was found to be granular and polypoid, and biopsy confirmed nasal rhinosporidiosis.

3. **Primary cutaneous type**: This type is uncommon [21]. Cutaneous lesions develop due to direct inoculation of organisms on the skin from its natural habitat. Lesions in the primary cutaneous type may be solitary or multiple. Sometimes secondary cutaneous lesions may also develop because of subsequent hematogenous dissemination [22].

Morphology of Cutaneous Lesions

Varied types of cutaneous lesions have been described (Fig. 6.1). The lesions are asymptomatic/painless. However, pain may be experienced when lesions are present in the sole [23].

Most common presentation of cutaneous rhinosporidiosis is warty papules/nodules with crusting and whitish spots on the surface. These whitish spots represent large sporangia [14].

It can also present as erythematous polypoid growth, skin-colored papule, subcutaneous nodules (solid or cystic), verrucous plaque, cutaneous horn, ulcers, cystic

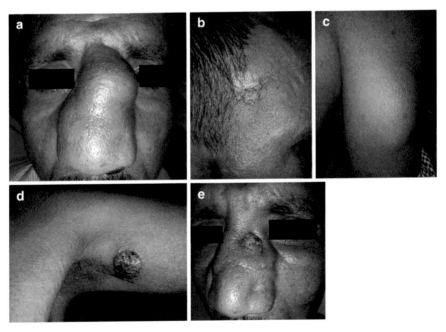

Fig. 6.1 Clinical images of a case of nasal rhinosporidiosis with disseminated cutaneous rhinosporidiosis showing multiple polymorphic cutaneous lesions. (**a**) Subcutaneous swelling over dorsum of nose. (**b**) Crusted plaque over right temporal region. (**c**) Subcutaneous swelling over right arm. (**d**) Pedunculated plaque with hemorrhagic crust over left axillary region. (**e**) recurrence of verrucous plaque over dorsum of nose after surgical excision

swelling, ecthymatoid lesions, furunculoid lesions, and nail changes (onycholysis, thinning, discoloration, and perforation of nail plate) [8, 12–19].

Rarely, the genitourinary system is also involved. Lesions can involve the penis, scrotum, urethra, vulva, and vagina [24]. The lesion can present as a polypoidal mass in fossa navicularis or penile shaft or glans penis [24], pedunculated swelling at the external urethral meatus [15], a painful bleeding nodule in labia minora [25], and pedunculated polypoid vaginal growth [26, 27].

The mode of infection in genitourinary rhinosporidiosis could be due to the inoculation of the organism using contaminated stones for mopping up residual drops of urine or autoinoculation by an infected fingernail or direct inoculation of spores in traumatized mucosa while bathing in contaminated stagnant water [5, 24]. The role of sexual transmission is controversial. However, Symmers described a case of vulval rhinosporidiosis where her male sexual partner had urethral rhinosporidiosis [25].

Sometimes polymorphic lesions are seen in a patient. For example, Kumari et al. described a case of disseminated cutaneous rhinosporidiosis with nasal rhinosporidiosis, with polymorphic cutaneous lesions in the form of a subcutaneous nodule, verrucous plaque, granulomatous growth, furunculoid lesions, and cutaneous horn-like lesions [17].

Complications

Cutaneous lesions bleed with trauma. Osteolysis of the underlying bone can be seen in subcutaneous lesions [11, 28]. Like recurrences in upper respiratory tract rhinosporidiosis, recurrence can be seen in cutaneous rhinosporidiosis [23]. Sometimes secondary cutaneous lesions may also develop because of subsequent hematogenous dissemination of primary cutaneous [22].

Differential Diagnosis

Lesions of cutaneous rhinosporidiosis mimic other common dermatoses. The differential diagnosis of various morphological variants are:

- **Warty lesions**: Verruca vulgaris, tuberculosis verrucosa cutis, pyogenic granuloma
- **Subcutaneous lesions**: Soft tissue sarcoma, chondrosarcoma [29], angiolipoma [30]
- **Ulcerated verrucous plaque**: Lupus vulgaris, subcutaneous mycoses [12]
- **Ulcerated lesions**: Basal cell carcinoma, squamous cell carcinoma
- **Genitourinary lesions**: Condyloma accuminata, donovanosis [14], penile malignancy [24], urethral caruncle [24]

Diagnosis

Clinical diagnosis of cutaneous rhinosporidiosis in contrast to nasal rhinosporidiosis is difficult. Few points favor the diagnosis of cutaneous rhinosporidiosis:

1. Patient presenting with cutaneous lesions with a present or past history of upper respiratory tract rhinosporidiosis.
2. Patient presenting with multiple cutaneous lesions of various morphology not fitting in other dermatoses, especially in an endemic area.
3. In case of suspicion, examine the lesions with a magnifying lens to look for whitish spots on the surface.

Once a presumptive diagnosis of cutaneous rhinosporidiosis is made, the following investigations will help in making a definitive diagnosis.

Investigations

- **Cytology**: Sample for cytological diagnosis can be taken by scraping superficial lesions or fine needle aspiration of deeper lesions, especially subcutaneous lesions [31]. For staining of smears, various special stains like Gomori methenamine silver, Periodic Acid-Schiff (PAS), mucicarmine, Grocott's stain, and Pappanicolaou's can be used. Examination of fine needle aspirate with 10% KOH is also diagnostic. In cytology, diagnosis is made by demonstrating sporangia in different stages of maturation and endospores admixed with inflammatory cells.
- **Histopathology**: The definitive diagnosis of rhinosporidiosis is made by histopathology [5]. Biopsy reveals a hyperplastic epithelium with a chronic inflammatory cell infiltrate composed of plasma cells, lymphocytes, and foreign body giant cells. Characteristic sporangia in various stages of maturation are seen as globular cysts of various sizes (50–1000 μm in diameter) lined by a well-defined wall containing numerous endospores of 5–10 μm.
- **Other investigations**: The cutaneous lesion in rhinosporidiosis may be an early sign of dissemination [12]. Investigations to rule out the involvement of other systems should be done, which includes blood counts, liver and renal function tests, X-rays of the chest and involved body part (especially in case of subcutaneous lesions to rule out underlying bone involvement), ultrasonography of the abdomen, computed tomography (to see the extent of the lesion, underlying bone and internal organ involvement).

Treatment

Total surgical removal of the lesion with diathermy coagulation of the base is the treatment of choice. Sometimes, wide local excision or partial amputation of the involved part is also required in case of extensive lesions [11]. The role of dapsone is controversial. However, it can be given as an adjunct to surgery as it may arrest the maturation of sporangia and accelerate degenerative changes in them.

References

1. Forsyth WL. Rhinosporidium Kinealyi. Lancet. 1924;1:951–2.
2. Ghorpade A. Giant cutaneous rhinosporidiosis. J Eur Acad Dermatol Venereol. 2006;20:88–9.
3. Acharya PV, Gupta RL, Darbari BS. Cutaneous rhinosporidiosis. Indian J Dermatol Venereol Leprol. 1973;39:22–5.
4. Arseculeratne SN, Arseculeratne G. Dermatological aspects of rhinosporidiosis. Exp Rev Dermatol. 2013;8:83–92.
5. Arseculeratne SN. Recent advances in rhinosporidiosis and *Rhinosporidium seeberi*. Indian J Med Microbiol. 2002;20:119–31.
6. Karunaratne WAE. The pathology of rhinosporidiosis. J Path Bact. 1934;XLII:193–202.
7. Sirka CS, Dash G, Pradhan S, Baisakh M. Cutaneous rhinosporidiosis presenting as cutaneous horn and verrucous plaque. Indian Dermatol Online J. 2019;10:178–9.
8. Nath AK, Madana J, Yolmo D, D'Souza M. Disseminated rhinosporidiosis with unusual involvement of the nail apparatus. Clin Exp Dermatol. 2009;34:e886–8.
9. Rajam RV, Viswanathan GC. Rhinosporidiosis: a study with a report of a fatal case with systemic dissemination. Ind J Surg. 1955;17:269–98.
10. Arseculeratne SN, Panabokke RG, Atapattu DN. Lymphadenitis, trans-epidermal elimination and unusual histopathology in human rhinosporidiosis. Mycopathologia. 2002;52:57–69.
11. Bandyopadhyay SN, Das S, Majhi TK, Bandyopadhyay G, Roy D. Disseminated rhinosporidiosis. J Laryngol Otol. 2013;127:1020–4.
12. Shenoy MM, Girisha BS, Bhandari SK, Peter R. Cutaneous rhinosporidiosis. Indian J Dermatol Venereol Leprol. 2007;73:179–81. https://doi.org/10.4103/0378-6323.32742.
13. Ghorpade A. Polymorphic ecthymatoid dermosporidiosis. Indian J Dermatol Venereol Leprol. 2008;74:298.
14. Thappa DM, Venkatesan S, Sirka CS, Jaisankar TJ. Gopalkrishnan, Ratnakar C. disseminated cutaneous rhinosporidiosis. J Dermatol. 1998;25:527–32.
15. Salim T, Komu F. Varied presentations of cutaneous rhinosporidiosis: a report of three cases. Indian J Dermatol. 2016;61:209–12.
16. Prasad K, Veena S, Permi HS, Teerthanath S, Shetty KP, Shetty JP. Disseminated cutaneous rhinosporidiosis. J Lab Physicians. 2010;2:44–6.
17. Kumari R, Nath AK, Rajalakshmi R, Adityan B, Thappa DM. Disseminated cutaneous rhinosporidiosis: varied morphological appearances on the skin. Indian J Dermatol Venereol Leprol. 2009;75:68–71.
18. Sen S, Agrawal W, Das S, Nayak PS. Disseminated cutaneous rhinosporidiosis: revisited. Indian J Dermatol. 2020;65:204–7.
19. Prabha N, Arora R, Chhabra N, Joseph W, Singh VY, Satpute SS, Nagarkar NM. Disseminated cutaneous Rhinosporidiosis. Skinmed. 2018;16:63–5.
20. Date A, Ramakrishna B, Lee VN, Sundararaj GD. Tumoral rhinosporidiosis. Histopathology. 1995;27:288–90.

21. Hadke NS, Baruah MC. Primary cutaneous rhinosporidiosis. Indian J Dermatol Leprol Venereol. 1990;56:61–3.
22. Nayak S, Rout TK, Acharjya B, Patra MK. Subcutaneous rhinosporidiosis. Indian J Dermatol. 2008;53:41–3.
23. Yesudian P. Cutaneous rhinosporidiosis mimicking verruca vulgaris. Int J Dermatol. 1998;27:47–8.
24. Pal DK, Moulik D, Chowdhury MK. Genitourinary rhinosporidiosis. Indian J Urol. 2008;24:419–21.
25. Symmers WS. Deep-seated fungal infections currently seen in the histopathological service of a medical school laboratory in Britain. Am J Clin Pathol. 1966;46:514–37.
26. Nair S, Hannah P. Rhinosporidiosis of vagina: a case report. J Trop Med Hyg. 1987;90:329.
27. Jahan S, Haque MA, Nessa F, Begum A, Hasan AH, Sen S, Huq MH. Vaginal rhinosporidiosis: a case report. Mymensingh Med J. 2014;23(3):572–4.
28. Adiga BK, Singh N, Arora VK, Bhatia A, Jain AK. Rhinosporidiosis. Report of a case with an unusual presentation with bony involvement. Acta Cytol. 1997;41:889–91.
29. Anjunwala P, Teissera DA, Dissanaike AS. Rhinosporidiosis presenting with two soft tissue tumors followed by dissemination. Pathology. 1999;31:57–8.
30. Tolat SN, Gokhale NR, Belgaumkar VA, Pradhan SN, Birud NR. Disseminated cutaneous rhinosporidiomas in an immunocompetent male. Indian J Dermatol Venereol Leprol. 2007;73:343–5.
31. Pal S, Chakrabarti S, Biswas BK, Sinha R, Rakshit A, Das PC. Cytodiagnosis of extra-nasal rhinosporidiosis: a study of 16 cases from endemic area. J Lab Physicians. 2014;6:80–3.

Clinical Presentation: Musculoskeletal Spectrum

Bikram Kar, Harshal Sakale, and Alok C. Agrawal

Rhinosporidiosis, first described by Guillermo Seeber in Buenos Aires, in Argentina, a rare chronic granulomatous disease endemic in some areas of Asia, such as central and south India and Shrilanka, with reported incidence in the America, Europe and Africa [1]. Rhinosporidiosis, a chronic and localized infection of the mucus membranes and the lesions present clinically as polypoid, friable soft masses (may be pedunculated) of the nose, throat, ear, conjunctiva, lips, uvula, palate, trachea, larynx, vagina, penis. The probable mode of infection from the natural aquatic habitat of Rhinosporidium seeberi is through the traumatized epithelium ('transepithelial infection') most commonly in nasal sites [2]. The etiological agent is Rhinosporidium seeberi, whose taxonomy has been debated in the last decades since the microoganism is intractable to islaolation and microbiological culture [3]. A detailed history of bathing habits and occupational exposure to stagnant water helps to reach at the clinical diagnosis, while histopathological examination of the excised mass confirms it [4–7]. Recurrence, dissemination in anatomically close sites and local secondary bacterial infections are the most frequent complications. Various modes of spread have been documented by several workers including; (i) auto-inoculation through spillage of endospores from polyps after trauma or surgery, (ii) hematogenous dissemination to distant sites, (iii) lymphatic routes, and (iv) sexual [8]. In extermely rare cases, rhinosporidiosis affects muscles and bone with peculiar presentation what we encountered.

B. Kar (✉) · H. Sakale · A. C. Agrawal
Department of Orthopedics, AIIMS, Raipur, India

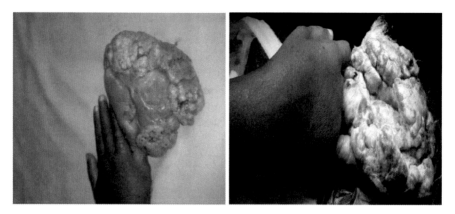

Figs. 7.1 and 7.2 Ulcerating and fungating mass arising from little finger and swelling and ulcer around the elbow

Clinical Presentation

Case 1

A 35-year-old woman presented with a 5-month history of swelling and an ulcerating and fungating mass in the anteromedial aspect of the right forearm and right little finger. There was serosanguinous foul smelling discharge from the swelling, which bled on touch. The mass was $9 \times 7 \times 5$ cm in dimension over right little finger, firm, friable, and multilobulated, with a delineated margin and the swelling was $6 \times 6 \times 4$ cm in dimension over right forearm near elbow (Figs. 7.1 and 7.2). There was no pain over the swelling and no fever. The patient also had multiple masses over face, abdomen, and back (Fig. 7.3). The nose and oral cavities did not reveal any lesions. The patient had a history of nasal rhinosporidiosis in her childhood for which she had been operated. The serological test for human immunodeficiency virus was negative. Radiography revealed a soft tissue shadow involving areas around right elbow and middle and distal phalanx of right little finger involving distal interphalangeal joint (Fig. 7.4). This case was managed with ray amputation of right little finger from the shaft of fifth metacarpal and excision of swelling from subcutaneous plane right forearm along with other cutaneous lesions (Figs. 7.5 and 7.6). Histopathology report showed sporangia of various shapes and sizes representing different stages of disease.

Case 2

A 23-year-old farmer from Raipur, India presented with 1-year history of progressive swelling over posteromedial aspect of the left thigh and proximal leg (Fig. 7.7). Swelling was painful and caused hindrance in the movement of leg. There was no history of trauma or significant weight loss.

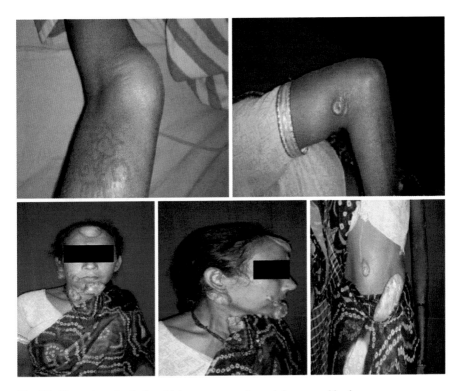

Fig. 7.3 The patient also had multiple masses over face, abdomen, and back

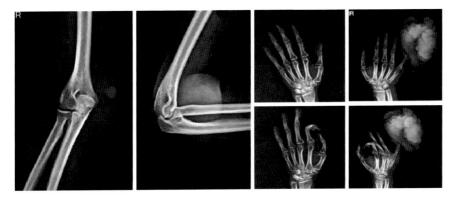

Fig. 7.4 X-ray of elbow and hand showing the soft tissue shadow

Patient was investigated and a venous color Doppler was performed which showed a large lobulated thick-walled multiseptated cystic lesion involving postero-medial aspect of the lower third of left thigh and upper half of left calf in the subcutaneous plane. CT peripheral angiogram showed a complex cystic lesion with peripheral enhancement in sartorius and gastrocnemius muscle. MRI left thigh and

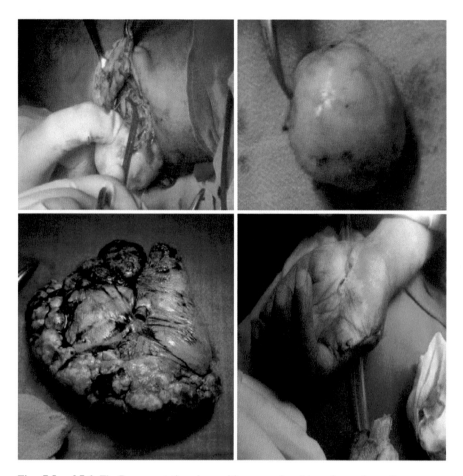

Figs. 7.5 and 7.6 The Ray amputation along with mass and excision of mass from elbow

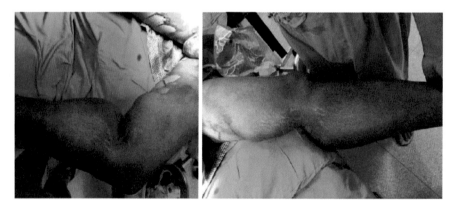

Fig. 7.7 Swelling over posteromedial aspect of the left thigh and proximal leg

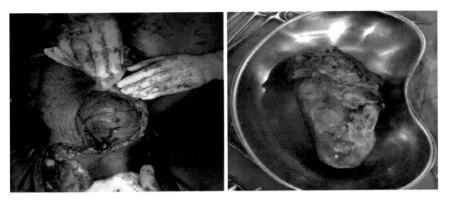

Fig. 7.8 Excision of swelling by extended posteromedial approach to proximal tibia and knee

left leg showed a well-defined heterogeneous signal intensity lesion at distal sarto-rius muscle along with medial compartment of the thigh and another similar lesion in superficial plane at popliteal fossa and upper calf region (Fig. 7.8). FNAC showed only clusters of neutrophils.

Diagnosis was confirmed by truecut core biopsy which showed fibromuscular tissue with numerous variable-sized thick-walled sporangia containing endospores in a background of chronic mixed inflammatory infiltrate comprising predominantly of lymphocyte and plasma cells. There was no evidence of malignancy in the sec-tions examined. Patient was counseled for surgery and a marginal excision of the mass performed by an extended posterior approach to thigh and knee.

Case 3

A 28-year-old farmer, on examination had non-tender, hard, fixed, non-pulsating swelling of size 10 × 5 cm over his right shoulder (Fig. 7.9) with overlying skin hyperpigmented and ulcerated anteriorly. An expansile, destructive lesion involving the lateral end of the right clavicle with soft tissue extension was visible. The clini-coradiological impression was of a primary bone tumor. No mucocutaneous lesions were seen.

Histopathological examination of the lesion revealed many sporangia and spores with the presence of lymphocytes and multinucleated giant cells. PAS stained smear showed many sporangia and spores along with giant cells suggestive of rhinosporidiosis.

All these cases were given dapsone for 6 months. They are on regular follow-up and are doing well.

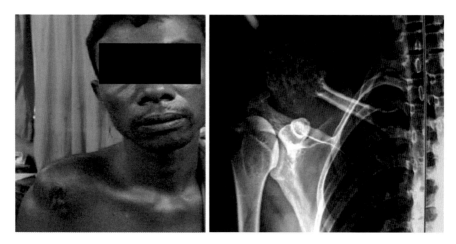

Fig. 7.9 Swelling over the shoulder at Acromioclavicular joint, X-ray shows, an expansile, destructive lesion involving the lateral end of the right clavicle with soft tissue extension

References

1. Karunaratne WA. Rhinosporidiosis in man. London: Athlone Press; 1964. p. 14–8.
2. Franca GV Jr, Gomes CC, Sakano E, Altermani AM, Shimizu LT. Nasal rhinosporidiosis in children. J Pedatr (Rio J). 1994;70:299–301.
3. Ahulwalia KB. New interpretation in rhinosporidiosis, enigmatic disease of the last 9 decades. J Submicrosc Cytolpathol. 1992;24:109–14.
4. Arseculeratne SN, Sumathipala S, Eriyagama NB. Patterns of rhinosporidiosis in Sri Lanka: comparison with international data. Southeast Asian J Trop Med Public Health. 2010;41(1):175–91.
5. Herr RA, Ajello L, Lepp PW, et al. Phylogenetic analysis of Rhinosporidium seeberi‖s 18S small subunit ribosomal DNA groups this pathogen among members of the protoctistan mesomycetozoea class. J Clin Microbiol. 1999;37:2750–4.
6. Venkatachalam VP, Anand N, Bhooshan O. Rhinosporidiosis: its varied presentations. Indian J Otolaryngol Head Neck Surg. 2007;59:142–4.
7. Capoor MR, Khanna G, et al. Rhinosporidiosis in Delhi, case series from a non-endemic area and mini review. Mycopathologica. 2008;168:89–94.
8. Adiga BK, Singh N, Arora VK, Bhatia A, Jain AK. Rhinosporidiosis. Report of a case with an unusual presentation with bony involvement. Acta Cytol. 1997;41:889–91.

Investigations and Diagnosis

Satish Satpute, Rupa Mehta, and Nitin M. Nagarkar

Diagnosis is mainly based on proper history, clinical examination, endoscopy, and radiological studies. In history, some baseline information makes it easy to approach for a diagnosis like nasal obstruction with epistaxis sometimes, bathing in pond water, history of previous surgery.

On clinical examination, Rhinosporidiosis masses are pink, painless, sessile or pedunculated with studded whitish yellow spores giving a typical strawberry like appearance. Infections of up to 30 years in duration have been reported. The main effects are discomfort when the lesion becomes large enough to obstruct a passage or puts pressure on nerves or vascular tracts. Symptoms vary according to the stage of development and site of infection [1, 2]. The infection produces a slow growing mass that degenerates into polyps. Endoscopically, the polyps are seen as pink to purple, friable, with gray, white, or yellow sporangia on their surface [3, 4]. Endoscopically we can also assess the site of origin and extent of mass.

Radiological evaluation is often required to delineate the extent of the lesion and the status of underlying structures. Many of these patients have undergone multiple previous surgeries, and hence, radiological assessment of deep-seated lesion in the nose and nasopharynx is essential to plan further surgery. The role of imaging in rhinosporidiosis is to evaluate the number of lesions, the location, and extent of disease, surrounding bone involvement, nasolacrimal duct involvement, and any associated complications. In cases of laryngeal and tracheobronchial involvement, CT helps in detecting the location of disease, extent of airway obstruction, and associated complications like airway obstruction, consolidation, and volume loss. On CT, rhinosporidiosis is commonly seen as a homogenously enhancing lobulated lesion in the inferior nasal cavity, extending into the vestibule anteriorly and through the choana into the nasopharynx posteriorly with erosion/rarefaction of the inferior turbinate. Multiple sites of involvement may be seen in cases with disseminated disease [5].

S. Satpute (✉) · R. Mehta · N. M. Nagarkar
Department of ENT and Head Neck Surgery, AIIMS, Raipur, India

© The Author(s), under exclusive license to Springer Nature Singapore Pte Ltd. 2022
N. M. Nagarkar, R. Mehta (eds.), *Rhinosporidiosis*,
https://doi.org/10.1007/978-981-16-8508-8_8

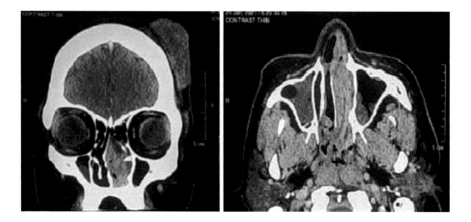

The gold standard for diagnosis is histopathological examination. Histologic microscopic examination reveals multifocal hyperplasia and ulceration on the mucosa, hyperplastic epithelium mainly within the mucosae of lamina propria, highly vascularized with fibromyxomatous connective tissue, a large number of R. seeberi with variable morphology within juvenile and mature sporangia may be seen by PAS and Mayer's Mucicarmin stain. Sometimes, mild hyperemia, mild multifocal hemorrhage suggestive of vascular invasion, necrotic focal areas on the submucosa or occasionally mild multifocal hemosiderosis may also be present. Inflammed nasal mucosa can be infiltrated with neutrophils (polymorphonuclear cells), eosinophils, lymphocytes, plasma cells (plasmocytes), mastocytes, giant cells, and histiocytes along with edema and numerous fungal sporangiospores inside the sporangium.

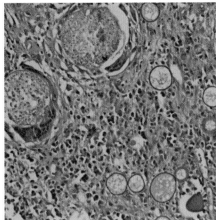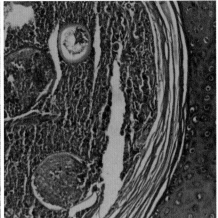

Sporangium size may range from 10 to 180 μm in diameter, enclosing sporangiospores of approximately 2 to 5 μm size or may vary often. The mature sporangia came out through the epithelial surface and release many endospores into the nasal exudates. Numerous neutrophils are present surrounding the free endospores while chronic inflammatory cells including macrophages, giant cells, and lymphocytes form a major part of fibro-myxomatous or fibrous stroma. In the stroma, giant cells may occur within sporangia also with prominent fibrosis mainly in non-respiratory locations of the body. In one clinicopathological study of 34 cases of rhinosporidiosis, generally, a lymphoplasmacytic response was observed in all cases. Polymorphonuclear leukocytic response is mostly observed at the site of rupture of sporangia. Epithelioid cell granulomatous and giant cell response were observed in 47% of cases. Transepithelial migration of sporangia was observed in 76% of cases [6].

Host Immune Response

Though in patients of rhinosporidiosis, anti-rhinosporidial antibodies are present in high titers but unlike other fungal or mycotic infections, Splendore-Hoeppli phenomenon is absent. It indicates by absence of any antibody-mediated eosinophilic deposition around rhinosporidial bodies in the host system. Studies project that cell-mediated immune response is activated but simultaneously with the immuno-suppression or with evidence of immune deviation means a switch from CMI to HI also takes place; from activation of CD4+ Th-0 cells, production of CD4+ Th-2 cells begin probably mediated by cytokines toward the production of anti-rhinosporidial antibodies [2–4]. R. seeberi evokes immune mechanism in humans, still it evades from host immunity through various suggested mechanisms. R. seeberi sporangia have a very thick outer wall that encompasses the antigenic structures inside so there is less chance for antibodies to act over it [5]. When there is destruction of the wall there is exposure of these antigens. This phenomenon is called as antigen sequestration. Herr et al. (1999b) reported that R. seeberi possesses the ability to vary their antigenic structures, and suggested that there is emergence of new antigenic structures when new sporangia emerge [6]. R. seeberi also causes immune suppression. Other mechanisms like immune distraction and immune deviation are also suggested for this pathogen [7].

References

1. Rhinosporidiosis. http://www.emedicine.com/med/topic2029.htm. Accessed 26 Apr 2002.
2. Rhinosporidiosis. http://www.doctorfungus.org/mycoses/human/other/rhinosporidiosis.htm. Accessed 26 Apr 2002.
3. Strickland GT. Hunter's tropical medicine. Philadelphia, PA: WB Saunders; 1984. p. 447.
4. Rippon JW. Medical mycology. 2nd ed. Philadelphia, PA: WB Saunders; 1982. p. 325–33.
5. Prabhu SM, et al. Imaging features of rhinosporidiosis 218. Indian J Radiol Imag. 2013 Aug;23(3):212–8.
6. Makannavar J, Chavan S. Rhinosporidiosis—a clinicopathological study of 34 cases. Ind J Pathol Microbiol. 2001;44(1):17.
7. Chitravel V, Sundararaj V, Subramanian S, Kumaresan M, Kunjithapadam S. Cell mediated immune response in human cases of rhinosporidiosis. Sabouraudia. 1981;19:135–42. https://doi.org/10.1080/00362178185380201.

Treatment of Rhinosporidiosis

Ripu Daman Arora, Nitin M. Nagarkar, and Megha Chandran

Rhinosporidiosis is quite an enigmatic disease which despite having been known to us for over a century, is confusing medical professionals all over the globe with its many unresolved characteristics starting from taxonomy to treatment. While its varied presentations, affected sites, modes of spread, etc. have been many a time elusive, surgeons have also found the treatment rather challenging due to its lack of proven conservative or medical management options and high recurrence rates.

Management of rhinosporidiosis is equally challenging as other aspects of the disease.

The most important factors of concern are recurrence, Immunology by pathogen, Incomplete excision Intraoperative contamination of adjacent tissues or cells with rending endospores.

Medical Management

The definitive treatment in case of Rhinosporidiosis is always surgical excision and any drug therapy tried or introduced is only an adjuvant to surgery.

Medical management for Rhinosporidiosis has been under trial for many years, but most drugs have been found futile. In an article published in 1936 by Allen and Dave [1] based on their study of 60 cases, they mention the use of Antimony compounds like Neostiban and Fouadin as adjuvant medical therapy for rhinosporidiosis but without proven effect. Trivalent and pentavalent antimony compounds were mainly used in the treatment of leishmaniasis and act by mechanism of prodrug action and host immune activation, but have not been proven to be useful in Rhinosporidiosis.

R. D. Arora (✉) · N. M. Nagarkar · M. Chandran
Department of ENT and Head Neck Surgery, AIIMS, Raipur, India
e-mail: director@aiimsraipur.edu.in

N. M. Nagarkar, R. Mehta (eds.), *Rhinosporidiosis*,
https://doi.org/10.1007/978-981-16-8508-8_9

Amphotericin B (a broad-spectrum antifungal agent) is another drug tried and found ineffective. In an article by Janardhanan et al. [2], they discuss a case report where a recurrent disseminated rhinosporidiosis patient was put on Amphotericin-B 1.5 mg/kg/day for 6 weeks owing to multiple recurrences while on dapsone therapy and surgery. Although a mild decrease in the size of lesions was noted while on treatment, the therapy was found to be ineffective both in cure and in recurrence.

The most useful and promising drug in rhinosporidiosis treatment is oral dapsone, which has been found to be useful as an adjuvant therapy in preventing recurrence as per a few case reports. Dapsone (4,4 diamino diphenyl sulphone) supposedly acts by the mechanism of arrest of sporangia and promotion of fibrosis within stroma [3, 4], thereby preventing recurrence. A study on microscopic findings in rhinosporidiosis [4] after dapsone therapy showed that after dapsone therapy in rhinosporidiosis, the organism showed accelerated degenerative changes and augmented host immune responses. It could therefore be expected that presurgical Dapsone would minimize both the hemorrhage by its promotion of fibrosis, as well as preventing the colonization and infection of new sites after the release of endospores from the surgically traumatized polyps [5].

A research article published in the *International Journal of Otorhinolaryngology Head Neck Surgery* [6] gives a crossectional study of 50 cases of rhinosporidiosis, where all patients were given postoperative dapsone therapy at a dosage of 2 mg/kg/day for a duration of 6 months. Only 4 patients showed recurrence and required resurgery. Many surgeons recommend a 1-year daily dose therapy of dapsone post-surgery.

Few articles also mention the use of postoperative adjuvant multidrug regimens of systemic drugs [7] like ketoconazole, cycloserin, along with dapsone in treatment of disseminated rhinosporidiosis.

Eight antimicrobial agents have been found to be effective anti-rhinosporidial therapeutic agents in order of decreasing potency: imidocarb diproprionate, diminazine aceturate, cycloserine, dapsone, trimethoprim-sulfadiazine, ketoconazole, sodium stibogluconate, and amphotericin B.[5]

Surgical Management

The definitive management of Rhinosporidiosis is surgical excision. Wide local excision with cauterization of the base [7] is the treatment of choice (Fig. 9.1), which has been improved over the years by the use of endoscopy and powered instruments. Currently, endoscopic excision of mass with cauterization of base is the treatment of choice for rhinosporidiosis excision.

Initially in earlier times, the removal was done by means of snare [1, 8] (hot or cold). But it was found that this was notorious for recurrence due to incomplete removal and multiplication of lesions due to fresh abrasions. The high recurrence rates in earlier times may be due to lack of endoscopic assistance and cauterization.

Fig. 9.1 Electrocautry in
Rhinosporidosis

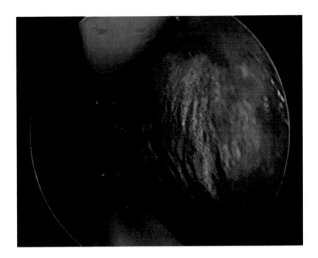

The employment of endoscopy and electric cautery for the destruction of surrounding infected mucosa was recognized to be effective in preventing recurrence.

Recently, the use of other powered instruments has been implemented including coblators and debriders for better and more complete disease clearance.

Coblation helps in complete resection of lesion with minimal bleeding and minimal damage to normal mucosa. It is a radiofrequency that penetrates tissues only up to 100 micrometer depth [9]. Its temperature also does not exceed 60 degree Celsius and also has a constant cooling effect due to simultaneous irrigation [10]. Coblation system can be a promising new tool in the surgical resection of recurrent rhinosporidiosis. It may also decrease the chances of reoccurrence due to very little contamination of the surrounding areas by preventing autoinoculation. Its novel design of the wand can help to remove the difficult-to-reach areas like posterior part of septum, around eustachian tube opening (Fig. 9.2).

Microdebriders have also been used for the completion of excision and residual disease clearance. The microdebrider is a powered rotary shaving device with continuous suction often used during sinus surgery. While the use of a microdebrider will not reduce the risk of bleeding, continuous suction allows your surgeons' vision of the surgical site to remain clear for much longer periods of time. Thus reduces the overall surgical time required to perform surgery Advantage being removal of broad base residual stocks followed by coagulating base although theoretically more risk of adjacent tissue dissemination (Fig. 9.3).

Laser is a relatively new tool that has come up as a safe adjunct in rhinosporidiosis surgery. It can be used for effective cauterization of surface attachments for recurrence prevention and hemostasis. Potassium Titanyl Phosphate (KTP) 352 and CO_2 lasers have been used in excision of rhinosporidial mass [11, 12]. Lasers can be considered superior to diathermy owing to their non-contact coagulation that causes minimum diseased tissue seedling and their dramatic reduction in bleeding.

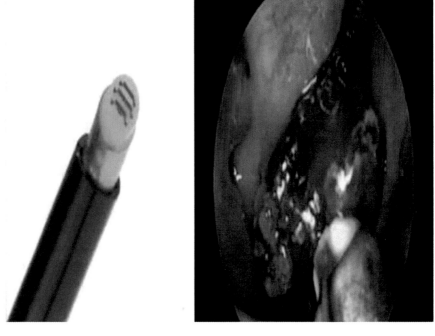

Fig. 9.2 Cobalator in Rhinosporidosis

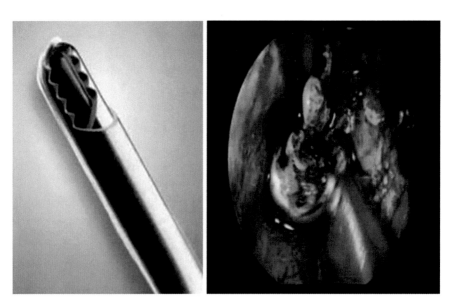

Fig. 9.3 Microdebrider in Rhinosporidosis

Conclusion

Rhinosporidiosis continue to challenge surgeons all around with diagnostic and treatment challenges. Even though treatment is fixed at a well-performed surgical excision with complete disease clearance, the focus needs to be on new and improved methods of excision and advancements directed at decreased recurrence with a special emphasis on the use of powered instruments like coblators and Laser. There is also a need to have more trials on adjuvant medical therapy that adds on effectively to surgery.

References

1. Allen FRWK, Dave ML. The treatment of Rhinosporidiosis in man based on the study of sixty cases. Ind Med Gaz. 1936 Jul;71(7):376–95.
2. Janardhanan J, Patole S, Varghese L, Rupa V, Tirkey AJ, Varghese GM. Elusive treatment for human rhinosporidiosis. Int J Infect Dis. 2016 Jul;48:3–4.
3. Das A, Das AK. Endoscopic excision of recurrent Rhinosporidiosis. Med J Armed Forces India. 2008 Jan;64(1):76–7.
4. Venkateswaran S, Date A, Job A, Mathan M. Light and electron microscopic findings in rhinosporidiosis after dapsone therapy. Tropical Med Int Health. 1997 Dec;2(12):1128–32.
5. Arseculeratne SN. Chemotherapy of rhinosporidiosis: a review. J Infect Dis Antimicrob Agents. 2009;26:21–7.
6. Shariff MA. A clinicopathological study of rhinosporidiosis in a tertiary care hospital. Int J Otorhinolaryngol Head Neck Surg. 2018 Jun 23;4(4):981.
7. George L, Dincy P, Chopra M, Agarwala M, Maheswaran S, Deodhar D, et al. Novel multidrug therapy for disseminated rhinosporidiosis, refractory to dapsone—case report. Trop Dr. 2013 Jul;43(3):110–2.
8. Singh I, Phogat D. Recurrent rhinosporidiosis: a case report. JOtolaryngol ENT Res. 2018 Nov 1;10(5):298–300.
9. Rachmanidou A, Modayil PC. Coblation resection of paediatric laryngeal papilloma. J Laryngol Otol. 2011 Aug;125(8):873–6.
10. Khan I, Gogia S, Agarwal A, Swaroop A. Recurrent Rhinosporidiosis: Coblation assisted surgical resection—a novel approach in management. Case Rep Otolaryngol. 2014;2014:1–4.
11. Swain S, Sahu A. An unusual presentation of rhinosporidiosis. Indian J Health Sci Biomed Res. 2021;14(1):156.
12. Kameswaran M, Kumar RS, Murali S, Raghunandhan S, Jacob J. KTP-532 laser in the management of rhinosporidiosis. Indian J Otolaryngol Head Neck Surg. 2005 Oct;57(4):298–300.

Pharmacological Aspects of Rhinosporidiosis

Pranav Sheth, Nitin Gaikwad, and Suryaprakash Dhaneria

Introduction

Rhinosporidiosis is a tropical disease caused by the organism *Rhinosporidium seeberi*, a lower aquatic fungus. It is a chronic granulomatous infectious disease characterised by large friable polyps in the nose (most common site), conjunctiva and occasionally in ears, larynx, bronchus and genitalia. Stagnant water is the main source of infection as spores are inhaled while taking bath in contaminated ponds and rivers.

Surgical excision is the main line of management for Rhinosporidiosis. A definite pharmacological therapy is not yet available for this disease. There are challenges to test the efficacy of antimicrobial agents against the causative organism, *Rhinosporidium seeberi*. *R. seebri* is difficult to cultivate in vitro and hence, in vitro methods based on multiplication of organisms cannot be used to assess the efficacy of drugs. The modified MTT-reduction method has been used to assess the anti-rhinosporidial activity of various drugs. However, in vitro results of anti-rhinosporidial activity of many drugs were not extrapolated clinically. Less clinical effectiveness may be attributed to the pharmacokinetic properties and poor penetration of drug into the lesion.

Various pharmacological agents such as dapsone, cycloserine, ketoconazole, amphotericin B, sulfadiazine-trimethoprim and sodium stibogluconate have been used in the treatment of Rhinosporidiosis with limited success. The pharmacological interventions that have been tried can be further classified into pre-surgical, post-surgical and entirely pharmacological management. In addition, interventions can be categorised as systemic therapy or topical therapy [1].

P. Sheth · N. Gaikwad (✉) · S. Dhaneria
Department of Pharmacology, AIIMS, Raipur, India
e-mail: nitingaikwad2707@aiimsraipur.edu.in

N. M. Nagarkar, R. Mehta (eds.), *Rhinosporidiosis*,
https://doi.org/10.1007/978-981-16-8508-8_10

83

Dapsone

It is the only drug that has demonstrated clinical efficacy against *R. Seeberi* in a few cases. Dapsone has been used alone or in combination with other agents in multi-drug therapy. The pharmacological details and account of this drug with reference to its use in the treatment of Rhinosporidiosis based on published literature is given in Tables 10.1 and 10.2, respectively. Table 10.3 shows the summary of case reports of use of dapsone in the treatment of Rhinosporidiosis.

In addition to the above case reports, several other case reports are available that have shown mixed outcomes after dapsone use [11–16]. However, in many of these case reports, dose and duration of dapsone and objective outcome were not mentioned.

Pre-Surgical and Post-Surgical Role of Dapsone

One of the serious complications of surgery in nasal and nasopharyngeal Rhinosporidiosis is profuse intraoperative haemorrhage due to high vascularity of the growths at these sites. The literature suggests that pre-surgical use of dapsone may arrest the disease process and minimise haemorrhage by promoting fibrosis and resolution of infection. It may also prevent the colonisation and infection of new sites due to release of endospores from surgically traumatised polyps [1].

Surgical excision of rhinosporidial tissue results in colonisation of normal mucosae by released endospores from the site of excision. Dapsone has been used post-surgically in most of the cases and few case reports suggest that recurrences have been minimised or prevented.

Table 10.1 Pharmacological details of Dapsone

Class of drug	Anti-leprotic drug; sulphonamide moiety
Important adverse drug reactions	Gastrointestinal ADRs—Anorexia, nausea, vomiting Dermatological ADRs—Skin rashes, phototoxicity, fixed drug eruptions, exfoliative dermatitis, toxic epidermal necrolysis, Stevens-Johnson syndrome Other ADRs—Bone marrow depression, Haemolytic anaemia, Methaemoglobinaemia, Agranulocytosis, Peripheral Neuropathy
Precautions	Avoid in patients allergic to sulphonamides, G-6PD deficiency patients, patients with severe anaemia Perform regular blood counts

Table 10.2 Pharmacological details of dapsone with reference to its role in the treatment of Rhinosporidiosis

Probable mechanism of action	Arrests the maturation of the sporangia and promotes fibrosis in the stroma
Route of administration used	Oral
Dose used in the treatment	50–200 mg per day Most commonly used dose—100 mg once daily
Duration of treatment	16 weeks to 24 months Most commonly used duration of treatment—6 months to 12 months

Table 10.3 Use of dapsone in the treatment of Rhinosporidiosis: Summary of case reports

Sr. No.	Lesion	Dapsone use	Outcome	References
1	Non-disseminated with multisite involvement in the head and neck	Without surgery 100 mg OD for 6 months	Favourable—Disease free at 1-year follow-up	K Devaraja, Prem Sagar, Chirom Amit Singh et al. [2]
2	Nasal	Without surgery 100 mg OD for 1 year	Favourable histopathological changes (degenerative changes in sporangia with loss of cytoplasmic material) in electron microscopy in biopsies taken after 10–12 weeks of dapsone therapy	S Venkateswaran, A Date, A Job et al. [3]
3	Parotid duct	With minimal invasive surgery Initially, 100 mg twice daily for 6 months, 200 mg daily for next 6 months	Favourable—At 16 months follow-up—No recurrence	Santanu Sarkar, Soumyajyoti Panja, Arghya Bandyopadhyay et al. [4]
4	Disseminated Rhinosporidiosis	Without surgery 100 mg once daily for 1 year	Favourable light and electron microscopy histopathological changes at 36 weeks (Maturation arrest of sporangia with an acceleration of degenerative changes) Disappearance of lesions at 1 year follow-up	A Job, S Venkateswaran, M Mathan et al. [5]
5	Lateral pharyngeal wall	Without surgery 100 mg BD for 1 year	Favourable—No recurrence at the end of 1 year follow-up	Vishnu Prasad, Vijendra S Shenoy, Raghvendra A Rao et al. [6]

(continued)

Table 10.3 (continued)

Sr. No.	Lesion	Dapsone use	Outcome	References
6	Lacrimal sac	Surgical excision 100 mg per day for 6 days a week for 6 months	Favourable—No recurrence at the end of 6 months follow-up	Sandip Kanti Basu, Jayanta Bain, Kuntal Maity et al. [7]
7	Nasal and nasopharyngeal	With surgical excision 100 mg once daily for 1 year	Dapsone + Surgery Group Partly favourable At the end of 3 years—No recurrence in 20 cases and recurrence in 8 cases with comparatively smaller growth and patients were asymptomatic. None required repeat surgery Only Surgery group At the end of 3 years—no recurrence in 2 cases, recurrence in 27 cases. Repeat surgery required in 27 cases.	Krishnan Nair [8] Comparative study—Surgery + Dapsone vs only surgery
8	Naso-sinal	Past history of use of dapsone for 1 year after partial excisional polypectomy Complete excision	Unfavourable—Recurrence Complete surgical excision—no recurrence at 1 year follow-up	Gawahir M Ali, Wael Goravey, Samir A Al Hyassat et al. [9]
9	Primary disseminated lesions over trunk and extremities	Without surgery 100 mg OD for 2 months	Unfavourable with single drug Drug stopped due to haemolytic anaemia. Patient shifted to multi-drug therapy (MDT) composed of cycloserine, ketoconazole, liposomal amphotericin B Outcome of MDT—Most lesions disappeared and decreased reasonably in size after 5 months of MDT	Ritwik Ghosh, Subharga Mondal, Dipayan Roy et al. [10]

Other Drugs Used

In addition to dapsone, the following drugs have shown some efficacy in in-vitro studies and few of them were used in management as multi-drug therapy. The pharmacological details of these drugs are depicted in Table 10.4.

In addition, sodium stibogluconate has also shown in vitro activity against the organism. However, literature related to its use in clinical practice is lacking. The granulomatous lesion of Rhinosporidiosis is surrounded by barriers to penetration of drugs such as oedema, haemorrhage, cell infiltration, cystic spaces, fibrosis and down-growth of squamous epithelia that surround the sporangia. Many drugs which have shown activity against organisms in in-vitro studies were not or less effective clinically. These differences in response may be attributed to poor penetration of drugs due to above-mentioned barriers or pharmacokinetic properties of drugs.

Role of Multi-Drug Therapy

In many case reports, the patients not responsive to dapsone or those who had recurrence after dapsone use, multi-drug therapy (MDT) has been tried. The clinical effectiveness of MDT in Rhinosporidiosis has been postulated due to their endospore static activity. The summary of case reports of the use of MDT in the treatment of Rhinosporidiosis is depicted in Table 10.5.

Table 10.4 Pharmacological details of other drugs used in the treatment of Rhinosporidiosis

Sr. No.	Drugs	Class of drug	Important ADRs
1	Ketoconazole	Antifungal drug; Imidazole group	Nausea, vomiting, anorexia, skin rash, pruritis, headache, hair loss, menstrual irregularity, gynaecomastia, reduced libido, impotence
2	Liposomal Amphotericin B	Antifungal drug; Polyene antibiotics	ADRs due to prolonged use—Nephrotoxicity, hypokalaemia, hypomagnesemia, infusion-related ADRs—fever, chills, muscle spasms, vomiting, headache, hypotension To be avoided in patients with renal failure or receiving concomitant nephrotoxic drugs
3	Cycloserine	Antitubercular drugs	Neurotoxic ADRs—headache, sedation, tremors, vertigo, confusion, nervousness, dysarthria, convulsions, suicidal tendency To be avoided in neuropsychiatric patients
4	Trimethoprim-Sulphadiazine	Sulphonamide	Skin rashes, toxic epidermal necrosis, Steven's Johnson syndrome, haemolytic anaemia, crystalluria Macrocytic anaemia, methaemoglobinaemia and haemolysis To be avoided in patients allergic to sulphonamides, patients with G-6PD deficiency

Table 10.5 Use of multi-drug therapy in the treatment of Rhinosporidiosis: Summary of Case Reports

MDT	Site	Outcome	Reference
Liposomal Amphotericin B 3 mg/kg IV once a day + Ketoconazole 400 mg BD + Cycloserine 250 mg for 5 months	Disseminated Rhinosporidiosis— Trunk and extremities	Disappearance of lesions and decrease in size of lesions	Ritwik Ghosh, Subhargha Mondal, Dipayan Roy et al. [10]
Cycloserine 250 mg TDS + Dapsone 100 mg OD + Ketoconazole 400 mg BD for 1 year	Disseminated Rhinosporidiosis— Trunk and extremities	Cutaneous lesions and subcutaneous nodules reduced in size No recurrence of mucosal lesions	Leni George, Peter Dincy, Manu Chopra et al. [17]
Cycloserine 250 mg TDS + Dapsone 100 mg OD + Ketoconazole 400 mg BD	Conjunctival Rhinosporidiosis	Favourable response— reduction in inflammatory response	Deepa John, Satheesh S. T. Selvin, Aparna Irodi et al. [18]

Drugs Used Topically

S Bhomaj et al. reported the topical use of 0.15% amphotericin B for treatment of peripheral keratitis caused by *Rhinosporidium seeberi*. In this case report, the complete resolution of ocular infection was observed and nasal polyp was removed surgically [19].

Conclusion

Rhinosporidiosis is a communicable disease caused by the organism *Rhinosporidium seeberi*. Surgical management is the mainstay of treatment in cases of Rhinosporidiosis. Many drugs have been tested for use in Rhinosporidiosis but the results have been mixed with some case reports claiming substantial improvement while others showing little improvement or recurrence of disease. Dapsone has been the most widely used drug. Apart from dapsone, multi-drug therapies have also been tried with some success.

References

1. Arseculeratne SN. Chemotherapy of Rhinosporidiosis: a review. J Infect Dis Antimicrob Agents. 2009;26:21–7.
2. Devaraja K, Sagar P, Singh CA, Kumar R. Non disseminated rhinosporidiosis with multisite involvement in the head and neck. Ear Nose Throat J 2018 Sep;97(9):E15-E17. https://doi.org/10.1177/014556131809700904. PMID: 30273436.
3. Venkateswaran S, Date A, Job A, Mathan M. Light and electron microscopic findings in rhinosporidiosis after dapsone therapy. Tropical Med Int Health 1997 Dec;2(12):1128–1132. https://doi.org/10.1046/j.1365-3156.1997.d01-212.x. PMID: 9438467.
4. Sarkar S, Panja S, Bandyopadhyay A, Roy S, Kumar S. Rhinosporidiosis of parotid duct presenting as consecutive bilateral facial swelling: a rare case report and literature review. J Clin Diagn Res. 2016 Mar;10(3):PD14–6. https://doi.org/10.7860/JCDR/2016/17633.7455. Epub 2016 Mar 1. PMID: 27134935; PMCID: PMC4843320.
5. Job A, Venkateswaran S, Mathan M, Krishnaswami H, Raman R. Medical therapy of rhinosporidiosis with dapsone. J Laryngol Otol 1993 Sep;107(9):809–812. https://doi.org/10.1017/s002221510012448x. PMID: 8228595.
6. Prasad V, Shenoy VS, Rao RA, Kamath PM, Rao KS. Rhinosporidiosis: a chronic tropical disease in lateral Pharyngeal Wall. J Clin Diagn Res. 2015 May;9(5):MD01–2. https://doi.org/10.7860/JCDR/2015/11831.5951. Epub 2015 May 1. PMID: 26155503; PMCID: PMC4484095.
7. Basu SK, Bain J, Maity K, Chattopadhyay D, Baitalik D, Majumdar BK, Gupta V, Kumar A, Dalal BS, Malik A. Rhinosporidiosis of lacrimal sac: an interesting case of orbital swelling. J Nat Sci Biol Med. 2016 Jan–Jun;7(1):98–101. https://doi.org/10.4103/0976-9668.175102. PMID: 27003980; PMCID: PMC4780178.
8. Nair KK. Clinical trial of diaminodiphenylsulfone (DDS) in nasal and nasopharyngeal rhinosporidiosis. Laryngoscope 1979 Feb;89(2 Pt 1):291–295. https://doi.org/10.1288/00005537-197902000-00011. PMID: 423667.
9. Ali GM, Goravey W, Al Hyassat SA, Petkar M, Al Maslamani MA, Hadi HA. Recurrent nasopharyngeal rhinosporidiosis: case report from Qatar and review of the literature. IDCases 2020 Jul 3;21:e00901. https://doi.org/10.1016/j.idcr.2020.e00901. PMID: 32685372; PMCID: PMC7355714.
10. Ghosh R, Mondal S, Roy D, Ray A, Mandal A, Benito-León J. A case of primary disseminated rhinosporidiosis and dapsone-induced autoimmune hemolytic anemia: a therapeutic misadventure. IDCases. 2021 Mar 16;24:e01076. https://doi.org/10.1016/j.idcr.2021.e01076. PMID: 33816117; PMCID: PMC8010393.
11. Madana J, Yolmo D, Gopalakrishnan S, Saxena SK. Rhinosporidiosis of the upper airways and trachea. J Laryngol Otol 2010 Oct;124(10):1139–1141. https://doi.org/10.1017/S002221511000126X. Epub 2010 Jun 8. PMID: 20529389.
12. Pal DK, Mallick AA, Majhi TK, Biswas BK, Chowdhury MK. Rhinosporidiosis in Southwest Bengal. Trop Dr 2012 Jul;42(3):150–153. https://doi.org/10.1258/td.2012.120177. PMID: 22785543.
13. Janardhanan J, Patole S, Varghese L, Rupa V, Tirkey AJ, Varghese GM. Elusive treatment for human rhinosporidiosis. Int J Infect Dis 2016 Jul;48:3–4. https://doi.org/10.1016/j.ijid.2016.04.013. Epub 2016 Apr 21. PMID: 27109109.
14. Prasad K, Veena S, Permi HS, Teerthanath S, Shetty KP, Shetty JP. Disseminated cutaneous rhinosporidiosis. J Lab Physicians 2010 Jan;2(1):44–46. https://doi.org/10.4103/0974-2727.66706. PMID: 21814408; PMCID: PMC3147087.
15. Nerurkar NK, Bradoo RA, Joshi AA, Shah J, Tandon S. Lacrimal sac rhinosporidiosis: a case report. Am J Otolaryngol 2004 Nov–Dec;25(6):423–425. https://doi.org/10.1016/j.amjoto.2004.04.012. PMID: 15547812.
16. Madke B, Mahajan S, Kharkar V, Chikhalkar S, Khopkar U. Disseminated cutaneous with nasopharyngeal rhinosporidiosis: light microscopy changes following dapsone therapy. Australas

J Dermatol 2011 May;52(2):e4–e6. https://doi.org/10.1111/j.1440-0960.2010.00633.x. Epub 2010 Mar 31. PMID: 21605088.

17. George L, Dincy P, Chopra M, Agarwala M, Maheswaran S, Deodhar D, Rupali P, Thomas M, Pulimood S. Novel multidrug therapy for disseminated rhinosporidiosis, refractory to dapsone—case report. Trop Dr 2013 Jul;43(3):110–112. https://doi.org/10.1177/0049475513493414. PMID: 23796478.

18. John D, Selvin SST, Irodi A, Jacob P. Disseminated Rhinosporidiosis with conjunctival involvement in an immunocompromised patient. Middle East Afr J Ophthalmol. 2017 Jan–Mar;24(1):51–53. https://doi.org/10.4103/meajo.MEAJO_89_15. PMID: 28546693; PMCID: PMC5433129.

19. Bhomaj S, Das JC, Chaudhuri Z, Bansal RL, Sharma P. Rhinosporidiosis and peripheral keratitis. Ophthalmic Surg Lasers 2001 Jul–Aug;32(4):338–340. PMID: 11475404.

Pathological Aspects of Rhinosporidiosis

Amit Kumar Chowhan and Nighat Hussain

Introduction

Rhinosporidium seeberi is a hydrophilic microorganism, the causative agent of the disease Rhinosporidiosis [1]. The *R. seeberi* is basically a protist placed under class Mesomycetozoa while earlier it was confused between fungi, protozoan, and cyanobacterium [2, 3]. The favorable climate for growth of these pathogens is believed to be hot tropical climate, therefore, a higher percentage of cases have been recorded from India and Sri Lanka, although the cases are recorded worldwide. Apart from affecting humans, this disease is also found to affect animals like primates, primarily livestock. The stagnant contaminated water of pond, tanks, wells serve as a reservoir for the growth of these microorganisms [3]. Thus, the patients suffering from this infection often have a history of bathing or swimming in dirty static water or they are working near riverbanks, therefore, the pathogen gets transmitted from water [4]. The disease primarily affects the mucous membrane of nasopharynx. Apart from nasal cavity, the other sites of involvement are lips, palate, uvula, larynx, trachea, conjunctiva, bone, penis, and vagina [5]. The clinical specifications of this disease are tumor-like red to pink friable, sessile polypoid masses that result in the development of chronic inflammation [1]. Nasal obstruction, epistaxis, and mucopurulent rhinorrhea are the most common symptoms of this infection. The contagious spread between humans and animals is very rare in this disease [2]. The diagnosis part involves the histopathological examination of the excised mass to confirm the disease [4]. Microscopically, different stages of maturation of spores can be observed as the dormant spores grow in contact with the living tissue [6]. Treatment of choice for rhinosporidiosis is wide local excision and cauterization of the base [7].

A. K. Chowhan (✉) · N. Hussain
Department of Pathology and Laboratory Medicine, AIIMS, Raipur, India
e-mail: chowhanpath@aiimsraipur.edu.in; hussain.nighat@aiimsraipur.edu.in

N. M. Nagarkar, R. Mehta (eds.), *Rhinosporidiosis*,
https://doi.org/10.1007/978-981-16-8508-8_11

Epidemiology

Classification

Rhinosporidiosis disease has a history of long debate for its taxonomic classification. Guillermo Seeber from Buenos Aires in 1900 described the first case in a nasal polyp [6]. In the honor of G. Seeber, Ashworth named the pathogen Rhinosporidiosis seeberi, after finding out that the disease is caused by a fungus. The studies were done in 18S rDNA sequence-based PCR (polymerase chain reaction) and FISH (fluorescent in situ hybridization) show the similarity of R. seeberi with member of genus Dermocystidium, an aquatic protistan fish parasites of Icthyosporea clade [2]. Analysis of 18S rRNA gene suggests that this organism is not a fungus but rather is the first known human pathogen from a novel aquatic parasite branch located near the animal–fungal divergence in the phylogenetic tree [1]. Earlier the organism was confused between lower fungi group, protozoan, and cyanobacterium. Now, the causative agent *Rhinosporidium seeberi* is considered as protist classified under order class Mesomycetozoa. The organism cannot be well grown in artificial media and its life cycle has not yet been properly studied.

Life Cycle of Pathogen

The life cycle of *R. seeberi* is still unknown and cannot be cultured in the lab [1]. The different stages can be studied in histological sections. The pathogen is an endospore forming organism and its life cycle has two stages "Trophocyte" (7 microns) and "sporangium" (300 microns). The sporangium is a mature thick-walled cyst filled with numerous spores, which may be up to 12,000 in number. The developing sporangia are present deep inside, whereas fully developed sporangia acting as a source of spores are found on the external surface. The spores if released from the sporangia can start a new life cycle in the nearby tissue [2].

Host Immune Response

The sporangia being the antigen, have a thick outer layer, thus antibodies produced from host have less effect on it. When there is destruction of the wall with release of antigens through the thick outer layer, the phenomenon is called *sequestration.* *R. seeberi* generates host immunity and evades it by several different mechanisms and also causes immune suppression. Although high titers of anti-rhinosporidial antibodies are seen in patient, still Splendore-Hoeppli phenomenon is absent. The Splendore-Hoeppli phenomenon, i.e., antibody-mediated-eosinophilic deposition is usually seen around the fungal elements in mycotic infections. The switch from cell-mediated immunity to humoral immunity also takes place because of immune suppression or immune deviation. The activation of CD4+ Th-0 cells produces

CD4+ Th-2 cells mediated by cytokines and proceeds toward the production of anti-rhinosporidial antibodies [2, 8, 9].

Transmission / Pathogenesis

R. seeberi naturally occurs in contaminated water and dust particles harboring spores. Water and soil act as a reservoir for this pathogen. The cases are frequently reported from the communities living near swamp areas. The ocular form can be caused through transmission from dust fomites and through drinking water, abraded nasal mucosa may get the infection. The incubation period is very long. The direct transmission between humans and animals is not reported yet, but the transmission can occur through swimming in contaminated water, inhalation of dust particles, direct contact with the pathogen spores through aerosols or infected clothing [2]. Karunaratne [10] postulated that Rhinosporidium existed in a dimorphic state. In soil and water, it existed as a saprophyte, whereas as a yeast form after reaching tissues.

Location

Although the disease is reported worldwide, but majority of cases were reported from tropical and subtropical countries. More than 90% cases are reported from India, Sri Lanka, and Pakistan [6]. However, it also occurs in Africa, South America, the Middle East, and Europe [1]. Europe reported least number of cases. Due to the hot tropical climate, southern part of India is endemic to this disease. It is stated that the content of chloride, a potent inhibitor of microorganism growth, in endemic country, India, is very less when compared to Western countries [1]. Intercontinental immigration and frequent travel is one important cause of global spread of this disease [2].

Sites of Involvement

Apart from nasal cavity and nasopharynx, the other sites of involvement are lips, palate, uvula, conjunctiva, ocular mucous membrane, epiglottis, larynx, bronchi, trachea, rectum, urethra, and even the bone. Rarely involved sites are ears, buccal cavity, pharynx, anus, vulva, penis, scalp, and cutaneous tissue [5, 6].

Common and Atypical Presentation

Rhinosporidiosis disease symptoms changes according to the stages of the life cycle of pathogen. First, the small mass is formed which degenerates into friable polyps. The color of sporangia changes from white, yellow, gray, and pink to purple. The common presentation of the disease starts with epistaxis, discomfort, nasal obstruction, and then it forms mucopurulent rhinorrhea. The lesion causes pain by blocking the nasal passage or any other affected site and also pressure is created on the neighboring nerves and vessels [2].

The atypical presentation of Rhinosporidiosis causes difficulty and confusion in diagnosis. The atypical presentation in the head and neck region is rare [5]. Generally, the atypical presentations in extra nasal sites which include conjunctiva, lacrimal sac, nasopharynx, oropharynx, skin, urethra, rectum, and rarely larynx and even bones, create diagnostic challenge. According to the study by Das et al., out of 114 patients, 16(14.04%) showed atypical presentation [7].

Rhinosporidiosis is more common in males, usually seen in young and middle-aged adults between 10 and 40 years [4].

Nasal Form

The pathogen or its spores after entering in body, targets the mucous membrane of the nasal cavity as it is the most common occurring form [2]. The presentation includes vascular, friable, sessile, or pedunculated polypoidal tumor-like masses in the affected site. The nasal obstruction and epistaxis are the common symptoms because of the friable and pendulous form of these lesions. The polyps can also present in palate, larynx, and nasopharynx [2].

Ocular Form

The ocular rhinosporidiosis consists of vascular, fleshy, soft, and polypoidal lesions. The affected sites are lacrimal sac, conjunctiva, sclera, and lids, in order of frequency. In India, the maximum cases reported are of palpebral conjunctiva [11].

Cutaneous Form

The cutaneous form is very rare and generally not present without the mucosal involvement. They present as asymptomatic warty growth. The treatment of cutaneous lesions should be done early to avoid extension of lesions or dissemination. Treatment of choice is surgical removal and diathermy excision, still recurrence is seen frequently [12].

Disseminated Form

The mode of dissemination, i.e., spread of *R. seeberi* throughout the body is reported in both affected person and animals. *R. seeberi* pathogen can disseminate to different regions of the body but, mainly it is documented in respiratory tract. The organism can also spread from respiratory tract to the limbs through hematogenous route. Although rare, anecdotal reports of involvement of regional lymph nodes are found in literature [13].

The disseminated forms are rare, which includes limbs, trunks, and viscera. If brain gets involved it will be fatal, also, if limbs get involved it will destruct the underlying bones [6]. The disseminated subcutaneous rhinosporidiosis is very rare. Disseminated rhinosporidiosis has been reported in a few cases of immunocompromised patients with conjunctiva and cutaneous involvement [14].

Das et al. [7] described a disseminated case with involvement of skin, subcutaneous tissue, radius bone, penis, urethra, with non-tender nodules on face and back in a long-standing primary lesion of nose.

Recurrent Rhinosporidiosis

Rhinosporidiosis shows recurrence when there is a decrease in anti-rhinosporidial cell-mediated immunity. Complete surgical excision is suggested to prevent recurrence. Along with the complete surgical excision, cauterization of the base is also suggested as the treatment. The recurrence rate is between 10% and 70% according to the literature reviews [9]. Incomplete removal of the mass leading to excessive bleeding or autoinoculation by surgical trauma leads to most of the recurrences. According to the study done by Das et al., two recurrent cases were reported both in nasopharynx, they found the complete clearance of the mass from nasopharynx is tough, because of multiple attachments and difficulty in exposure and instrumentations leading to endospores spillage in the surrounding mucosa during removal [6, 7].

Diagnosis

Sino nasal endoscopy is mentioned as a standard test to precisely assess nasal obstructive disease and it is considered necessary in all patients with nasal obstruction, also Computed Tomography scan (CT) of the nose and paranasal sinuses is the ideal imaging examination (gold standard) to study nasal and paranasal sinus diseases [15].

Microscopically, the organisms vary from small spores to mature thick-walled sporangia that contain numerous refractile endospores (Figs. 11.1 and 11.2). These are highlighted with periodic acid-Schiff, Gomorimethenamine silver and Mucicarmine stains (Figs. 11.3, 11.4 and 11.5).

Transepithelial migration is noted in some cases. The organisms usually induce a chronic inflammatory response comprising lymphocytes and plasma cells. Neutrophilic response is noted at the site of rupture. Giant cell reaction as well as granulomatous inflammation composed of epitheloid cells and giant cells may also be observed.

Fig. 11.1 Photomicrograph illustrating squamous epithelial lining with mature, immature, and collapsed sporangia surrounded by inflammatory cell infiltrate (H&E, ×10)

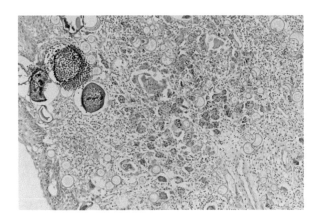

Fig. 11.2 Photomicrograph illustrating double-walled sporangia with numerous refractile endospores (H&E, ×40)

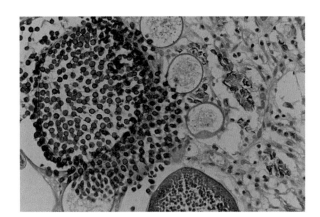

Fig. 11.3 Photomicrograph illustrating double-walled sporangia with numerous endospores stained pink (PAS, ×40)

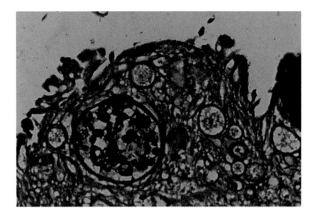

Fig. 11.4 Photomicrograph illustrating double-walled sporangia with numerous endospores stained black (GMS, ×40)

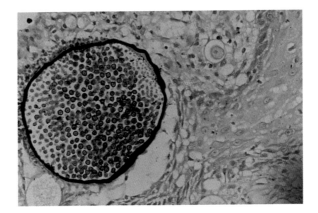

Fig. 11.5 Photomicrograph illustrating sporangium with hyaline wall filled with numerous sporangiospores (Mucicarmine, ×40)

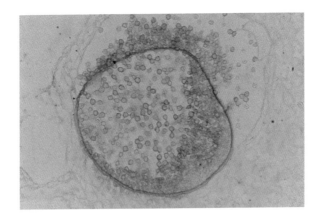

References

1. Seray T. Rhinosporidium seeberi: is it a fungi or parasite? Turkiye Parazitol Dergisi. 2020;44:258–60.
2. Tiwari R, Karthik K, Dhama K, Shabbir MZ, Khurana SK. Rhinosporidiosis: a riddled disease of man and animals. Adv Anim Vet Sci. 2015;3:54–63.
3. Gupta RK, Singh BP, Singh BR. Rhinosporidiosis in Central India: a cross-sectional study from a tertiary care hospital in Chhattisgarh. Trop Parasitol. 2020;10:120–3.
4. Karthikeyan P, Vijayasundaram S, Pulimoottil D. A retrospective epidemiological study of Rhinosporidiosis in a rural tertiary care Centre in Pondicherry. J Clin Diagn Res. 2016;10:4–8.
5. Saha J, Basu AJ, Sen I, Sinha R, Bhandari AK, Mondal S. Atypical presentations of rhinosporidiosis: a clinical dilemma? Indian J Otolaryngol Head Neck Surg. 2011;63:243–6.
6. Sinha A, Phukan JP, Bandyopadhyay G, Sengupta S, Bose K, Mondal RK, et al. Clinicopathological study of rhinosporidiosis with special reference to cytodiagnosis. J Cytol. 2012;29:246–9.
7. Das C, Das S, Chatterjee P, Bandhopadhyay SN. Series of atypical Rhinosporidiosis: our experience in Western part of West Bengal. Indian J Otolaryngol Head Neck Surg. 2019;71:1863–70.

8. Jayasekera S, Arseculeratne SN, Atapattu DN, Kumarasiri R, Tilakaratne WM. Cell-mediated immune responses (CMIR) to Rhinosporidium seeberi in mice. Mycopathologia. 2001;152:69–79.
9. De Silva NR, HuegelHeino ADN, Arseculeratne SN, Kumarasiri R, Gunawardena S, Balasooriya P, et al. Cell-mediated immune responses in human rhinosporidiosis. Mycopathologia. 2001;152:59–68.
10. Karunaratne WA. Rhinosporidiosis in man. London: The Athlone Press; 1964.
11. Sood N, Agarwal MC, Gugnani H. Ocular rhinosporidiosis: a case report from Delhi. J Infect Dev Ctries. 2012;6:825–7.
12. Prasad K, Veena S, Permi HS, Teerthanath S, Shetty KP, Shetty JP. Disseminated cutaneous rhinosporidiosis. J Lab Physicians. 2010;2:44–6.
13. Arseculerantne SN. Recent advances in rhinosporidiosis and Rhinosporidium seeberi. Ind J Med Microbiol. 2002;20:119–31.
14. John D, Selvin S.T. S., Irodi A and Jacob P. Disseminated Rhinosporidiosis with conjunc-ticval involvement in an immunocompromised patient. Middle East Afr J Ophthalmol 2017;24:51–53.
15. Prakash M, Johnny JC. Rhinosporidiosis and the pond. J Pharm Bioallied Sci. 2015;7:S59–62.

Research Topics in Rhinosporidiosis

Rupa Mehta, Ambesh Singh, and Nitin M. Nagarkar

Rhinosporidium seeberi as a causative organism of rhinosporidiosis is well known for more than 100 years [1]. It has been recorded in around 70 countries. Still, so many uncleared enigmas persist regarding its microbiological characterization, spread, its relationship with immunity of individual and histopathology like detection of sporangia transdermally, pattern of cellular infiltration with variation in the affected cell with rhinosporidiosis. Rhinosporidium seeberi has so far neither been cultured in vitro. Apart from human beings, other domestic and wild animals, - cows, buffaloes, dogs, cats, horses, mules, ducks, and swans, have also been found to be affected.

There are many unexplained aspects of rhinosporidiosis which require further dedicated research in collaboration with all countries in which it is endemic.

On the top of the list is the position of the organism in the world of microbiology, whether it is a fungus, a protozoa, an algae, or something else?. It is now classified as part of the DRIP clade (Dermocystidium, Rosette agent, Icthyophonus, and Psoropermium), a group of fish parasites that flourish in hot and humid climate. Rhinosporidiosis seeberi is placed in order Dermocystida, previously orphaned aquatic microbes, located at the divergence between animals and fungi. Still there is no consensus regarding its taxonomic position. It defies Koch's postulates and has still not been cultured. It has not been produced experimentally in animals. Epidemiological studies suggest that the main natural habitat of R. seeberi is groundwater in ponds and lakes, or in soil that is contaminated with such water. Mode of spread, immunological reaction in the host following infection, immune status of the person which makes him more susceptible to have infection, reasons

R. Mehta (✉) · A. Singh · N. M. Nagarkar
Department of ENT and Head Neck Surgery, AIIMS, Raipur, India

N. M. Nagarkar, R. Mehta (eds.), *Rhinosporidiosis*,
https://doi.org/10.1007/978-981-16-8508-8_12

for endemicity in certain regions need to be clearly defined. Only a few people in the family or the locality having the same habits get the disease.

Climate conditions, stagnant water with its physicochemical property plays a vital role in its endemicity. Biodiversity of the ponds are different in endemic regions. Physiochemical properties of water in India and Sri Lanka are more in favor of rhinosporidium growth when compared to the West. Acidic pH, less sodium and chloride favors microorganism growth. It is a known fact that chlorine is a potent inhibitor of microorganism growth. It is to be determined if some public health measures, like chlorination, seggregating waterbodies for animal and human use can reduce the burden of the disease.

Rhinosporidiosis clearly has a definite relation to exposure to stagnant water/ contaminated pond bathing. It needs to be investigated if there a possible synergism between aquatic microorganisms and Rhinosporidium seeberi for the propagation of infection through stagnant water. It is well documented regarding the mode of infection by autoinoculation, hematogenous or lymphatic spread but it causes quite an uncertainty when it comes to explaining the infectivity of the disease. Not all/ only a few who are exposed are encountering the disease; its chronicity lasting for several years, all lead to a definite immunological pattern. But little is known about immune responses in human rhinosporidiosis which are responsible for predominant characteristics of disease like chronicity, recurrence, and dissemination, despite presence of high antibody titers.

Clinical features—Many unexplained clinical presentation features are there which require further elucidation. What may be the cause of increased incidence of rhinosporidiosis in "O" blood group individuals (about 70%)? [2]. Why lymph nodes are not involved? There is no recurrence following complete removal even if the patient lives in the same environment. There may be an immunological cause for non-recurrence. Are there any dietary factors involved? Do subtle unrecognized immunodeficiencies play a role?

Human leukocyte antigen type of the people in the endemic areas may be different when compared to the others which may explain the geographical variations.

Why nose and nasopharynx are commonly affected while sinuses are not involved.

Why oropharynx and skin are frequently involved but oral mucosa (buccal mucosa) is rarely involved?

How is nasolacrimal sac involved by the disease—retrograde from the nose or through the eyes? What is the mechanism of involvement of the parotid duct? Why submandibular gland is not involved ?

Why do few patients have distinct unifocal involvement while others have multifocal involvement? What factors make patients prone to have disseminated disease? What are the predisposing factors that make the patient susceptible to have multiple recurrences?

Diagnosis of the disease is mostly clinical and histopathological. Contrast enhanced Computed Tomography (CECT) scan of nose and PNS is the radiological investigation of choice in nasal rhinosporidiosis [3]. However, since there are no specific characteristic features, it is mainly used for surgical planning in recurrent disease (distorted anatomy due to previous surgical procedures).

Definitive treatment of choice is surgical (endoscopic) excision [4], or by using combined approach (open + endoscopic approach). There are challenges to test the efficacy of antimicrobial agents against the causative organism. Adjuvant Dapsone therapy (interferes with maturation of spores, thus preventing recurrence) can be used in patients with extensive disease with no G6 PD deficiency but results have been equivocal [5]. Few multi drug therapies have also been tried. Despite the disease being known for so many decades, no other drug has been found effective for the treatment. Due to a high rate of recurrence, long-term follow-up is indicated.

Conclusion

Still, research is required to say evidently regarding the natural habitat, chemical and physical properties of water, immunological aspect, chronicity, culture of the organism, newer drugs and newer surgical technologies for treatment so as to reduce the recurrence rates.

References

1. Arseculeratne SN. Recent advances in rhinosporidiosis and Rhinosporidium seeberi. Indian J Med Microbiol. 2002 Jul 1;20(3):119–31.
2. Kameswaran S, Lakshmanan M. Rhinosporidiosis. In: Kameswaran S, Kameswaran M, editors. ENT disorders in a tropical environment. Chennai: MERF Publications; 1999. p. 19–34.
3. Prabhu SM, et al. Imaging features of rhinosporidiosis on contrast CT. Indian J Radiol Imaging. 2013 Aug;23(3):212.
4. George L, Dincy P, Chopra M, Agarwala M, Maheswaran S, Deodhar D, et al. Novel multidrug therapy for disseminated rhinosporidiosis, refractory to dapsone—case report. Trop Doct. 2013 Jul;43(3):110–2.
5. Arseculeratne SN. Chemotherapy of rhinosporidiosis: a review. J Infect Dis Antimicrob Agents. 2009;26:21–7.